Praise for *The Winning Mindset that Saved My Life*

Tom Hulsey has always sought-out challenges, embraced their difficulties, and overcome them. This time, however, rather than seeking it out, the crushing emotional and physical challenge of confronting and finding a way to survive prostate cancer, both physically and emotionally, sought-out Tom.

In *The Winning Mindset That Saved My Life*, Tom shares deep, inspiring, and touching insights into the principles of personal resiliency which can help each of us address both the planned and unplanned challenges which are an inevitable part of life.

That Tom chose the challenge of completing the Ironman Triathlon World Championship Race in Kailua-Kona Hawaii, with its legendary heat, wind, and suffering, as the challenge with which to put the exclamation point on his survival, is both inspiring, and speaks volumes about Tom!

The Winning Mindset That Saved My Life is a deeply inspiring, insightful, must read for all of us who face challenges as we journey through life!

Bob Whitman
Chairman and Chief Executive Officer, FranklinCovey

Hearing a diagnosis of cancer can be terrifying and isolating. With *The Winning Mindset That Saved My Life*, Tom Hulsey elegantly describes how he navigated the fears and feelings he experienced after being diagnosed with prostate cancer at age 61. An elite IRONMAN athlete, Tom has sage advice for methods of managing the minefield of surviving the diagnosis, treatment, and survivorship of cancer using a positive mindset, relying on family and friends for support, eating a healthy diet and reducing stress, and educating oneself about the disease and treatment options. Tom Hulsey provides a roadmap to health in the face of cancer, and by extension shares his expansive view of living with cancer, and beyond. I recommend *The Winning Mindset That Saved My Life* for any cancer survivor and their loved ones. It is an engaging read that will give survivors hope for the future and a plan for now!

Kelvin A. Moses, MD, PhD, FACS
Assistant Professor of Urologic Surgery
Vanderbilt University Medical Center

Prostate cancer is a prevalent malignancy that touches the lives of many men. Though effective treatments are available, many of them can be associated with temporary and sometimes permanent morbidities. In THE WINNING MINDSET THAT SAVE MY LIFE, Mr. Hulsey shares inspiring and thoughtful reflections from his journey with prostate cancer. It is uplifting and full of great quotes and insights, and it will help many patients and their families who are facing this disease.

Ashley E. Ross, M.D., Ph.D.
Urologic Oncology
Texas Urology Specialists

Executive Medical Director
Mary Crowley Cancer Research

As a prostate cancer survivor, I can say every word in Tom Hulsey's book can be leaned on to help you in your fight. There are many choices you will be forced to make, your first and most important is to have an "I will beat this attitude!"

Reading Tom's book can help you set your sights on that goal. As I read it, many times he took me back to my personal battles and what carried me through to victory. Be informed!

Barry Davis
Anchor/Investigative Reporter
CBS/KENS 5

As a fellow cancer survivor, I was very thankful to have met Tom during my journey. His insights and honesty regarding his struggle with this horrible disease really helped me better understand the mindset I needed to make decisions and fight through my recovery.

I was equally impressed with his goal-setting and even more so, the amazing accomplishments; who competes in the IRONMAN - the hardest, most grueling competition of its kind months after surgery? Not many people, I can assure you. Few regular folks can even come close, present company included!

Then he shifts gears and passionately attacks the need for a cure - he now is getting prostate cancer on the radar of our government and insurance companies, while continuing to provide hope to those fighting this disease and those who have survived.

I am very thankful Tom came into my life at a time when I had way more questions than answers.

As Tom so famously says "Life is not a spectator sport!"

Dean Xeros
CEO, Principle Logistics Group

With Coach Tom's guidance, we were able to provide our sons a well-balanced hockey experience from their elementary years through high school. They were athletes, but also band members, and strong students. Tom worked to create a better HUMAN. He was not just about sports. He also cheered on their achievements in soccer, band, and academics . . . and he does so for both of our sons to this day. Learning to be mindful of life's options absolutely provided both of our sons with advantages that have transferred to every goal they have undertaken- in high school, college, and now grad school. Both of them have experienced success in the demanding Texas A&M Corps of Cadets. They don't focus what is not when circumstances become difficult . . . they build on what is. Thankfully, this was reemphasized in the Corps at A&M, as they were selected to guide underclassmen in their academic and leadership growth. Tom didn't simply develop hockey players. He developed LEADERS.

The Winning Mindset That Saved My Life allows readers to follow Tom's journey and challenges as he faced (and defeated!) prostate cancer, as well as to examine their own lives through personal reflection. It is a story of challenge, adversity . . . encouragement and victory.

Ann Fry
Hockey Mom & Teacher

Tom has done the prostate cancer community a true service by writing about his experiences, his passions, and his battle with prostate cancer. The challenges of prostate cancer almost always touch men by surprise and for men to take control of the situation and learn how to persevere is one of the most important issue that can occur in a patient's journey.

How does a patient know what to do? How does a patient know which doctor to seek? How do you engage with your physicians in making the best decisions for your case? All of these are critical questions, which are necessary for each and every patient to address. Finding the right support, finding the right competitive edge is always key to overcoming life's challenges. Tom shares his journey in an inspirational way and the hope is that patients everywhere will benefit from his experiences.

Oliver Sartor, M.D.
C.E. & Bernadine Laborde Professor for Cancer Research
Medical Director, Tulane Cancer Center
Assistant Dean for Oncology
Tulane Medical School

There are pitfalls in life. We all encounter them. What matters most is reaching out a hand to the next person who falls down and saying, "here, let me show you the way". *The Winning Mindset that Saved My Life* does just that. In 16 years as an advocate for cancer patients and a leader in the nonprofit industry, I have never met anyone with a more powerful positive mindset than Tom Hulsey. Tom's prostate cancer journey from diagnosis to Kona Ironman Triathlete to no quit advocacy leader inspires and paints a pathway to survive and thrive past life's most daunting challenges.

Jamie Bearse
Chief Executive Officer, ZERO The End of Prostate Cancer

There are certain people who make you a better person. Tom Hulsey is one of those people. Tom is one of the most inspirational people I have ever met, and his great desire to back is second to none. His energy and enthusiasm are evident in the substantial time he volunteers in helping cancer patients, his philanthropic work and is a humble servant and leader to everyone he meets.

I have known him personally and professionally for 25 plus years and he really has challenged me and inspired me. His mission (legacy) is to find a cure for cancer, as exemplified by his new book, *The Winning Mindset that Saved my Life*. Net profits from this book will be donated to cancer research. I admire Tom's candor and leveraging his story to "make a difference!"

You will find his message inspirational no matter where you are in life, facing a challenge or setting new goals, Tom can give you that little bit of extra encouragement we all need now and then.

Mary Anne (Wihbey) Davis
Peak Performance Solutions

Tom Hulsey's *The Winning Mindset That Saved My Life* is a compelling portrait of one man's successful battle with what scares all of us post-50 men . . . a cancer diagnosis. Tom's journey is poignant, vivid, and told from the heart. In my 35+ years managing people and players in professional sports, I can attest and support Tom's thesis that it really is the mind . . . positive thinking and a powerful mental approach . . . that differentiates people and performance in most circumstances. A good read with positive lessons for all of us.

Jim Lites
President/CEO, Dallas Stars Hockey Club

Jack,

My journey has created a passion in me to help others battle cancer, including those close to cancer victims. I feel fortunate to have a mission to help others, to help them through the battles I survived. I've grown to appreciate the value of serving a greater cause than my own self-interest; making a positive impact on Humankind. If this book impacts just one person; that's my definition of success,

Life is not a spectator sport,

Jon

The Winning Mindset

that

Saved My Life

ISBN: 978-1-937-045-029

Front Cover: Tom Hulsey before the
2016 IRONMAN World Championship
Kailua-Kona, Hawaii

Back Cover: Tom Hulsey crossing the finish line at the
2016 IRONMAN World Championship
Kailua-Kona, Hawaii

Dedication

I dedicate this book to the memory of my friend, Bill Rollings. Bill lost his battle with prostate cancer May 13, 2013.

I also dedicate this book to the memory of my Urologist and confidant, Michael Gruber. Dr. Gruber died unexpectedly March 3, 2018.

Acknowledgments

I have many people to thank for the completion of this project. I want to express my sincere thanks and deep appreciation to Ann Lovett Baird for her superb assistance in helping me articulate my journey.

Thanks to the many friends who encouraged me to share my story in a book, including Todd Carter and Michael Conley.

Thanks to my urologist, Dr. Michael Gruber and the many health care professionals who restored me back to good health.

Thank you to Jan Klodner who helped turn my attitude around and realize that by setting goals, "Anything is possible."

Thank you to Jamie Bearse and ZERO – The End of Prostate Cancer, for giving me a purpose and enabling me to make a difference. Thanks to the hundreds of donors who shared my passion for making a difference by supporting my fund-raising.

Thanks to Willy Waks, James Mays, Nilo Castillo and Steve Zuehlke for "being there."

Thanks to my sponsors Cyber Defenses, Inc. and Vitality Sports Medicine.

Thanks to Dave Deschenes, Executive Director at the IRONMAN Foundation for your graciousness at Lake Placid and Kona.

Most of all, thank you to my wife, Lauren, who has patiently and pleasantly helped me keep at it throughout these many months of writing.

Foreword

There are many challenges in life. Some are self-determined or internal, such as running a marathon or achieving one's dreams of becoming a doctor, for example. Other challenges are thrown at us externally, such as financial hardship or being diagnosed with a life-threatening illness. Having the right mindset holds the key to overcoming these challenges. In *The Winning Mindset that Saved My Life* Tom Hulsey uses his battle with cancer as an illustration of how developing the right state of mind is crucial to succeed in overcoming both internal and external challenges.

Prior to his diagnosis of prostate cancer, Mr. Hulsey became a triathlon champion. He uses the same approaches to being a winning athlete as he does to overcoming the emotional and physical trials and tribulations of the diagnosis and treatment of prostate cancer. He discusses how his own traits of perseverance, overcoming fear, living intentionally, and knowing his options enabled him to proactively approach building a mindset and create a clear vision of where he wanted and needed to go with regard to accepting the diagnosis of cancer and the recovery from treatment. The right mindset takes courage and diligence. It takes a person out of their comfort zone. Mindset drives the choices a person makes and the habits they develop.

The Winning Mindset that Saved My Life elegantly and simply weaves together medicine, physiology and sports psychology with Mr. Hulsey's life experiences as a coach, instructor, athlete, and cancer survivor. Quotes and inspirational messages from world leaders, authors, and athletes are united with personal experience. He demonstrates that the skills and discipline required for a triathlon are the same skills and discipline that can be used to battle cancer or any other challenge in one's life. The book is organized in logical order starting with the ironman triathlon and his personal background. Thereafter, there is a detailed explanation of what having a winning mindset entails. The book closes with an optimistic assessment of how to grow and achieve further and tackle additional trials after an initial challenge is overcome. Woven into this is the story of surviving prostate cancer.

This is an inspirational journey and one that any patient with cancer or other life-threatening or life-altering obstacle should read and incorporate into their daily routines and rituals. I highly recommend it for my patients and my colleagues as every person confronts tribulations, impediments, and challenges that can be overcome with a winning mindset.

Mitchell Sokoloff, M.D., F.A.C.S.
Professor and Chair
Department of Urology
University of Massachusetts Medical School
UMass Memorial Health Care

Table of Contents

"A life is not important except in the impact it has

on other lives."

Jackie Robinson

Introduction

Why am I writing this book? Cancer took me by surprise. I have been a competitive athlete for as long as I can remember and have strived to maintain a healthy lifestyle. I've always had the attitude that I could compete in any sport or event that I chose to. That belief led me to compete in my first IRONMAN at Kona, Hawaii in 1986, the first of eleven IRONMANs that I have raced in my life.

The cancer diagnosis destroyed that belief. At first I didn't even want to fight the battle with cancer. I'm not here to brag, just to share my journey from despair at a cancer diagnosis to the victory of beating it.

My journey has created a passion in me to help others battle cancer, including those close to cancer victims. I fought my particular battle with prostate cancer, yet much of what I share here applies to other forms of cancer and life challenges. Filled with uncertainty and unpredictability, life's journey reminds me of my favorite Beatles' song, "The Long and Winding Road."

Gratefully, I had the skills and discipline required to prepare for and compete in IRONMAN competitions, because those very abilities helped me deal with cancer. In addition, my strong support group consisting of Lauren, my wife, Willy Waks, Steve Zuehlke, Jan Klodner, James Mays and Nilo Castillo, allowed me to stay focused when preparing for IRONMANs, and, in my battle with cancer. They encouraged me, and reminded me that I am a fighter and fighters don't quit.

I always say that an IRONMAN is a metaphor for life. You have your ups and downs, your challenges, unforeseen mishaps and fears that you power through. When life happens in an unexpected way, these same skills and disciplines help you deal with the curveballs in life.

Having said that, here's what I hope you will get out of this book:

- ☐ How to take control of and fight for your health
- ☐ How you and your caretakers can journey through the waters of illness
- ☐ Inspiration, courage and hope for whatever challenge you face
- ☐ The ability to look beyond today's circumstance in your life to embrace a life of purpose and meaning
- ☐ Perseverance and triumph over whatever life hands you

What is an IRONMAN?

To give you a feel for IRONMAN, here's a little history.

As quoted on the IRONMAN website,

"During an awards banquet for the Waikiki Swim Club, John Collins, a Naval Officer stationed in Hawaii, and his fellow athletes began debating which athletes were the fittest: swimmers, bikers, or runners. Later, he and his wife Judy, who had both participated in new competitions known as triathlons in San Diego, decided to combine three of the toughest existing endurance races on the island. On February 18, 1978, 15 competitors, including Collins, came to the shores of Waikiki to take on the first-ever IRONMAN challenge.

In 1980 founders John and Judy Collins gave ABC's Wide World of Sports permission to film the event, bringing worldwide recognition to IRONMAN. Only two years later, college student Julie Moss collapsed just yards from the IRONMAN World Championship finish line. Someone passed her at the finish line, but she didn't give up. She crawled to the finish line, unknowingly creating one of the most iconic moments in IRONMAN history.

With the recognition of the Physically Challenged Athletes in 1997, Australian John MacLean becomes the first athlete to power a hand cycle bike and wheelchair to an official IRONMAN World Championship finish. Today, hundreds of thousands of triathletes from around the world have challenged themselves to prove to friends, loved ones, and even themselves that "Anything is Possible". Have you been inspired to Become One?" [1]

An IRONMAN competition includes a 2.4-mile swim, 112-mile bike ride and 26.2-mile run.

Here's what journalist Eric Greene says of his experience at the Kona IRONMAN in 2016.

"The Kona race is notorious for being the most physically and mentally challenging course of the IRONMAN network. The leeward side of Hawaii's Big Island is a largely barren desert of lava fields, subject to strong winds, extreme heat, and drastic inclines between coastline and volcanoes. The lush tropical rainforest of Hawaiian stereotype does not live here, and the world's best endurance athletes are constantly humbled in the harsh environment. All competitors are well aware of the demands they face and you can feel their concern for days leading up to the main event.

The atmosphere in town underwent an ominous change on the eve of race day. People were panic training in the early morning darkness, others paced with their heads down through the day. You could feel how tense it was as silence consumed the evening. The following morning, the streets were full at 4:30 A.M. ahead of the starting gun as the sun appeared over the island's rugged, volcanic landscape. It was

---

[1] IRONMAN.com

cruel and unusual, and without a doubt the most intense and emotional sporting event I've ever witnessed."2

An IRONMAN is someone who completes the race in under 17 hours. This disciplined athlete can and will put in the work, overcome mental roadblocks, demonstrate the mental and physical stamina to keep on going when the body and the mind say, "I can't go on." This athlete takes on all challenges and overcomes. This person doesn't quit and truly believes that "Anything is possible".

No matter what you face in your life, remember, "Anything is possible"!

---

2 Eric Greene; FieldMag.com; *Why IRONMAN Matters — A first-timer's raw experience as a spectator of the World's biggest triathlon & Behind the scenes at Kona World Championships*.cite Eric Greene article

My Story

I have always made my health a priority. My parents influenced me from an early age. Mom always taught me to listen closely to my body. She taught me that the body uses pain to warn of something wrong, so I've always paid close attention to that. My Dad and my college roommate, Rex Horton, greatly influenced my commitment to a healthy lifestyle. Dad started jogging and swimming in the 1960s during the first running boom, influenced by the Father of Aerobics Dr. Ken Cooper. Rex, a Division 1 wrestler and cheerleader, practiced discipline in his diet and workouts. I saw the benefits of a healthy lifestyle in both men, up close and personal. Both had a huge impact on me, which led to my commitment to set an example and inspire others to live a healthy lifestyle.

My love of sports started with skating on the ponds of Wisconsin when I was five years old. I learned to play hockey and was pretty good at it, which eventually impacted my tennis game. My tennis coach told me to use the same swing with the tennis racket that I used with a hockey stick. I tried that and sure enough, it made a difference. I really liked tennis and worked hard at it. The work paid off and I found myself as one of the top tennis players on my high school team. In the 1980s, I discovered Triathlons and ultimately, the IRONMAN. Once I got into triathlon-type races, I was hooked.

My success in sports helped me create the mindset I needed for the discipline and lifestyle required to train for an IRONMAN. IRONMAN training requires a daily commitment to the training schedule to support the ultimate goal of competing in the race. Mindset is key to keep that training going, to run, swim or bike those miles on a day when you don't feel like it. I never had a triathlon coach. I trained by trial and error, just figuring out how to train and doing what seemed best, day in and day out.

Mindset impacts every part of life and everything that happens to you, good or bad. Mindset gives you a way of viewing the world and everything in it. We each need to decide how to live and what actions to take. That's why I have this motto: "Life is not a spectator sport." And yet, my success as an athlete gave me a false sense of invincibility. I developed an arrogant mindset. My cancer diagnosis changed all that.

Dreaded Words

"You have cancer."

In February 2015, on my 61st birthday I heard those dreaded words from my doctor. After 10 months of doctor visits because of elevated PSA levels, which continued to increase, a biopsy confirmed my fears. For ten months prior to the diagnosis, worry and dread dominated my thoughts and the possibilities of what would happen to me. This came on the heels of watching my long time friend Bill Rollings spend four years battling and ultimately losing his battle with cancer. I didn't want to end up like Bill. With every visit up to this point I grew more despondent and depressed. I didn't talk to anyone, outside of a few people like my wife, about my situation.

Anxiety filled my life and started to control me. My head spun in disbelief. My sense of success and the ability to deal with any challenge shattered. Often I thought, why me? Haven't I done everything right to stay healthy? I've always tried to inspire others to live a healthy lifestyle. Now I felt like a fraud, and ashamed to tell anyone I had cancer. I didn't even want to fight. I told my doctor I didn't even want to discuss the options.

Dealing with a cancer diagnosis alone and in secret proved a lonely place. If I had to do it over again, I'd have shared my situation with others sooner. I agonized for thirteen months after my diagnosis.

Support of Family and Friends

My family and close friends had a powerful impact on my attitude and mindset about cancer. I wanted to give up in the face of cancer and the arduous battle to beat it, but my wife reminded me of the fight I had in me. She helped me look beyond Bill Rollings' battle to my own life. With her help, I saw the importance of my life to those around me. My story could end differently than Bill's.

Several months after my diagnosis and some pep talks from Lauren, I confided in a close friend, Jan Klodner, a fellow FBI Citizens' Academy Alum. He helped pull me out of my depression and feeling of hopelessness. He inspired me to move from hopelessness to hopefulness by setting goals, to shift from the despair of my situation to the hope the future. Jan did not face a life-threatening illness, yet he applied what he did to recover from major surgery to inspire me out of my depressed state.

When I explained my situation and the cancer diagnosis with him, he shared how he had overcome his recent health challenge. Jan had double knee-replacement surgery, which requires a long and challenging recovery. In addition to being a busy and successful business owner, Jan has a passion for racquetball. He taught me that when life gives you adversity, set goals and never give up.

Jan made it his post-surgery goal to play racquetball in four months. By setting specific goals and keeping his ultimate target in front of him, he found himself back on the court in four months. He persevered, and continued ramping up his game until he played competitively six months after his surgery.

Jan's clarity of purpose to play racquetball competitively again gave him the drive to continue working at his game every day in spite of the challenges he faced with his recovery. Every day he had to make the decision to continue, to persevere, to look toward the future and follow his plan. Even though he might have felt like quitting on one day or another, he never did. He knew he had to keep going toward his goal no matter what.

Jan encouraged me to set goals to get beyond cancer. Knowing that I had a passion for IRONMAN, he reminded me of the IRONMAN motto, "anything is possible." Looking back, this advice contributed to saving my life. I was ready to give up. His advice emboldened me! At that point, my mindset started to shift and proved a pivotal point in my battle. Based on his encouragement, I set short, intermediate, and long-term goals, which shifted my focus from hopelessness to the future, beyond cancer. If Jan had not given me this encouragement, I might have given up before even starting the battle.

Ultimately, I had a Robotic Prostatectomy May 7th, 2015, National Prayer Day. This gave me a level of solace at a very scary and uncertain time in my life. I knew people were praying for me because of the peace and reassurance I had in my heart. Though the surgery saved my life, for me, the mindset shift came first. I felt such despair and depression about the thought of cancer and the battle against it, that I needed the mindset shift to even get to the operating table.

I found recovery extremely rough, both mentally and physically. Using a walker to get around humbled me. Other physical complications that come with recovering from this type of surgery meant I had to swallow my pride and focus on gratitude for being alive. I had always prided myself as ultra-fit and strong! This was not the picture after surgery.

I am grateful to have survived cancer and to have raced two IRONMANs since then. The skills and discipline required for IRONMAN are the same skills and discipline that I used in my cancer battle. I hope that my story and my journey can inspire you in any challenge you have in life, whether it's cancer, finances, loss of a loved one or loss of a meaningful relationship.

Mindset holds the key to overcoming life's challenges. The components of mindset that have served me my whole life include perseverance, overcoming fear, living intentionally, and knowing my options. All these helped prepare me for a battle I never thought I'd have to fight. For me, preparation for whatever happens in life also means looking at options when life doesn't happen the way you expect.

Reflective Questions

What life challenge do you face?

Who can help you in the challenge?

The Journey to IRONMAN

As I mentioned, I've been an athlete all my life. The pinnacle of my athletic life is the IRONMAN. I raced a total of eleven IRONMANs, nine prior to cancer and two after cancer. I tell you this to demonstrate how far I fell with my cancer diagnosis, and what I had to do to come back. My love of triathlons and the IRONMAN started in the 1980s, yet my love of sports and my journey there started long before that.

As I mentioned earlier, as a teenager, I loved hockey and tennis. By my junior year in high school, I started looking for an activity to complement hockey. I went out for the baseball team and got cut. So, I turned to tennis. I made it as the last man. Tennis is very hierarchical, so I was slotted on the number two doubles team. With my coach's advice to swing my tennis racket like a hockey stick, my tennis game soared. By my senior year, I was ranked as the number one singles player on the team.

My interest in a multi-sport like a triathlon began in 1983. I attended the World Championship Tennis (WCT) tournament at Reunion Arena in Dallas in the spring of 1983. This men's professional tennis tour included tennis greats like John McEnroe and Jimmy Connors. There, I picked up a brochure for a short-distance triathlon at nearby Lake Lavon. I wanted another physical endeavor, but found this intimidating. Friends insisted that triathlon was beyond my grasp. To me, this sport had appeal because it allowed me to train on my schedule.

I worked odd hours in Information Technology (IT), so training on the bike, in the pool and running trails to fit my schedule made a lot of sense. As a tennis player, I found it hard to find opponents during a weekday. As it turned out, I did not compete in that race in 1983. I listened to the naysayers and backed out. However, a true connection with multi-sport began. I never lost my intrigue with triathlon.

Fast forward, one year later, to the identical scenario at the WCT tournament. In spite of doubts from those around me, I entered the 1984 President's Triathlon at Lake Lavon. I felt motivated to prove people wrong. The race challenged me and I had a lot of takeaways from it. I found out that swimming in a lake with a lot of people around is a lot different than swimming in a pool. A triathlon swim is a contact sport with legs and arms ready to slap you from every direction. Next, I had that feeling in my legs of trying to run after cycling on a bike for twenty-one miles - yikes!

Somehow I finished and so began my love affair with triathlon. I completed more triathlons of varying distances in 1984 and 1985.

In 1985, I watched ABC's Wide World of Sports telecast of the 1985 IRONMAN, held in Hawaii. IRONMAN mesmerized me. Despite having never come close to doing any of the distances, I set a far-fetched goal of racing at the 1986 IRONMAN.

Before I even knew if they'd accept me as a participant at Kona in 1986, I started training with that goal in mind. I knew I had to totally commit to racing at Kona, and prepare mentally and physically to even have a chance to survive the heat of Hawaii and the race distances for swimming, cycling and running. The training regimen took focus, determination and consistent training day after day to prepare for this new type of race.

First, I had to run a marathon, so I ran the Dallas White Rock Marathon in December 1985. I had success there and my confidence started to build. The far-fetched goal of racing in an IRONMAN started to feel more reachable.

Since I had not competed in any qualifying races to qualify for Kona, I entered the lottery for the 1986 IRONMAN race. I knew the difficult odds of getting in, but I thought to myself, I'll never know if I can do it or not if I don't try. In April 1986, I received a postcard saying they had selected me for the October race! I didn't know whether to cry or laugh. With no books written about training, and no triathlon coaches, I found myself on my own. I trained by trial and error.

As former sponsor Mike Ramsey said about me, "He was like the rest of us back then. Go hard, go long and go again tomorrow."

I biked 100 miles for the first time six weeks prior to the IRONMAN at the Hotter-n-Hell Bike Rally in Wichita Falls, Texas. That gave my confidence a real boost, plus the heat in Wichita Falls is similar to the heat in the lava fields in Hawaii. Speaking of the heat, I did my run training in the late afternoon, the hottest time of the day in my home state of Texas to prepare for this great event. I knew what I needed to overcome to compete in and finish the race. This brutal training schedule taxed me physically, but it had the added benefit of conditioning my mind for a race that could last up to 17 hours.

Self-Absorbed Discipline

As much as I love triathlons and the associated discipline, anyone who has done it knows it as a selfish, self-absorbed activity. Very much an individual sport, it requires a significant investment of time. Everyone around you has to understand and support your commitment to training. Both my employer and health club supported this endeavor by sponsoring me. Zale Corp and Fitness Unlimited paid for my clothing, transportation, hotel and food.

People viewed me in one of two ways: Crazy because of the insane and seemingly unhealthy distances or admirable, because of my determination and grit. I had the vision and goal before me, and I let nothing get in the way of my training regimen.

My innate perseverance, mindset, ability to overcome fear and intentional lifestyle got me through my first IRONMAN. I kept working at building my endurance and strength. As it turns out the disciplines that got me through that first IRONMAN eventually saved my life when I had to battle cancer.

Mindset truly made me an IRONMAN and a cancer survivor. The right mindset supported those daily actions I needed to prepare for and complete IRONMAN competitions and to defeat cancer. For without a shift in mindset sparked by my conversation with Jan Klodner, I might have given in to depression and despair. I am grateful to the doctors and the surgery that ultimately saved my life, but I never would have even considered them if I did not have hope.

Reflective Questions

What lofty goal do you want to achieve?

What steps do you need to take to achieve that goal?

Choose Your Mindset

"All things are created twice; first mentally, then physically. The key to creativity is to begin with the end in mind, with a vision and a blueprint of the desired result."

Stephen R. Covey

The dictionary defines a mindset as a habitual or characteristic mental attitude that determines how you will interpret and respond to situations. An intentional act doesn't happen by accident. As Covey says, all things start with creation in the mind.

Developing the right mindset is crucial to succeed in anything. You must proactively approach building your mindset by creating a clear vision of where you want to go. These images of your goal create a strong pull toward the end-result.

As a triathlete, one of the biggest success factors of any race came from being in the right spot mentally. In every workout during the months leading up to a big race, I'd think about a part of the course and figure the best way to approach it to make race day a great day. I visualized the outcome I wanted to achieve.

Finding the right pace in a long race like IRONMAN comes from your mental game. The brain must make endless computations by taking in all the signals to determine whether you are maximizing a sustainable pace. At the same time, the brain assesses any pain signals that may require you to slow down, then, figures out if you are going as fast as you can without flaming out and not finishing.

It's complicated! You'll find many ways to get from the start to the finish. Over time, you'll find the one that works best for you, and that one will make you forget the possibility of an outcome other than crossing the finish line in time.

So many things can run through your mind during the race. Maybe fear sets in. You worry that you won't achieve your goal. No matter the scenario playing out in your mind, especially a negative one, you have to just shut off the internal chatter and race.

Discomfort is a byproduct of peak performance for any athlete. I learned to focus on something beyond the pain. I learned from more experienced athletes, how to deal with pain.

IRONMAN champion Mark Allen had a great strategy. Here's what he said.

"If all else failed, I would look around at where I was. Most of the time, it was a beautiful place, a vacation destination. Yes, even the stark lava of The Big Island of Hawaii is a paradise if looked at through the right lens. I had to forget that I was not feeling super at that moment. Remember how lucky I was to still be out there racing. I was doing something that most of humanity would not even consider!

I would remember key workouts I did getting ready for the race that had moments that were tough. I gained strength from that memory knowing that I made it through them. I had full access to the all the fitness that I stored up getting ready for the race. Finally, after working through these steps as I was racing, my focus was no longer blocked by negative chatter. I would start rising to a level that I never thought possible a moment earlier."[3]

Life is the same way isn't it? You will not have perfect days every day. Whether battling cancer, dealing with the loss of a loved one, or any of life's disappointments, you have to know life will never be perfect. You have to ride it out.

The devastation of a cancer diagnosis took my mind down a very negative track, and I don't mean to minimize the impact of a negative event in your life. Only to say that, to overcome that negative track starts with hope, and that you have to keep working through the process every day.

---

[3] https://blog.markallencoaching.com/big-race-mindset/

Turning your mind to the beauty around you, as Mark Allen described, can move you past a current feeling of discouragement. Thinking about what you are grateful for can move your thoughts in a totally different direction. Your attitude or mindset in anything is a choice.

When I heard my urologist say those three words, "You have cancer," I had to retune my mindset. As you saw earlier in my story, this did not come easily. I went through a process to overcome my fear and re-calibrate my mindset.

What is a Winning Mindset?

For me personally, perseverance, overcoming fear and living intentionally comprise the key components of a winning mindset. More than attitude, mindset goes deeper, to conviction of action and creating a habit of the mindset that wins. Mindset helps you through when circumstances challenge you. Mindset makes you a stronger person over time.

Mindset is so impacted by positive attitude. As a hockey coach, I wanted to impact kids with a positive attitude. For that reason, the following quote from a parent of some of the kids I coached means a lot to me. I coached three kids in the Warhoftig family. Here's what David Warhoftig had to say.

"One of the things that stands out most – and with all three of my kids – is that you told them how to be respectful and how to do things in a way that is positive, no matter what odds you face.

You have been an amazing guide for my children of what to do in life and how to do it the right way! I tell you all the time – and sincerely mean it – that you have made a difference and I really look up to you in how you go about living life."

The positive attitude doesn't mean that we don't look at something that needs change and address it. One of David's sons grew totally discouraged with hockey. I gave him exact instructions on what changes to make, and I did it with a positive attitude, far different from other coaches. Here's what David said.

"My middle child played his first season of hockey on an absolutely terrible house team and his experience from top to bottom was one of incredible frustration and disappointment. After that season he wanted to quit.

And after just a few minutes with you, that magic happened! You looked right at him, you held him when he needed it for difficult moves, you smiled, you laughed, and most of all you taught! You taught him that hockey can be fun and that there was so much more to the game and to the world than what he had experienced. Within a few months, you gave him the confidence that he needed and taught him to love the game."

I share this story only as a demonstration of the power of your mindset. Not only for you, but for those around you. Helping someone else improve their mindset gave me a boost too!

Do you have an Intentional Mindset?

Maybe you fear you won't achieve a goal you've had for a long time, or you feel like giving up on a dream that you've had for a long time. You must make the intentional choice to keep that dream in front of you to drive your mindset. You can keep your dream in front of you with pictures that represent achieving that dream. Post the pictures where you will see them every day. The pictures have an amazing impact on your mind. Maybe you want a different job and you need new skills. Write a resume that describes the future state and the skills and experience that you have. Having the end in mind drives your subconscious mind and your actions.

If your mindset produces negative chatter, you have to stop and re-direct what's playing in your mind, because your mind ultimately directs your actions, even when you don't realize it. That is not to say that you might not have a bad attitude one day. You just have to ride it out and not stay there. Ride it out and re-direct. A winning mindset allows you to push through the negative or down times to keep on going.

Keep going until you see the next step to take. And remember, those down times or circumstances in your life are temporary. That helps give a context for what you face and to move you away from fear, anguish and a negative attitude.

In the same way that Mark Allen looked around at his surroundings during an IRONMAN, you can list in your mind all you are grateful for. Research indicates that brain chemistry actually changes when you think about what you are grateful for. What a powerful tool to improve your mindset.

In an article on *psychologytoday.com*, Alex Korb, Ph.D. says this about brain chemistry and gratitude.

"The wide variety of effects that gratitude can have may seem surprising, but a direct look at the brain activity during gratitude yields some insight. The final study I'm going to share comes from the National Institutes of Health (NIH). NIH researchers examined blood flow in various brain regions while subjects summoned up feelings of gratitude (Zahn *et al,* 2009). They found that subjects who showed more gratitude overall had higher levels of activity in the hypothalamus. This is important because the hypothalamus controls a huge array of essential bodily functions, including eating, drinking and sleeping. It also has a huge influence on your metabolism and stress levels. From this evidence on brain activity it starts to become clear how improvements in gratitude could have such wide-ranging effects from increased exercise, and improved sleep to decreased depression and fewer aches and pains.

Furthermore, feelings of gratitude directly activated brain regions associated with the neurotransmitter dopamine. Dopamine feels good to get, which is why it's generally considered the 'reward' neurotransmitter. But dopamine is also almost as important in initiating action. That means increases in dopamine make you more likely to do the thing you just did. It's the brain saying, "Oh, do that again."

Gratitude can have such a powerful impact on your life because it engages your brain in a virtuous cycle. Your brain only has so much power to focus its attention. It cannot easily focus on both positive and negative stimuli. It is like a small child: easily distracted. Oh your tummy hurts? Here's a lollipop. So you lost your job? Isn't it wonderful we're having KFC for dinner? On top of that your brain loves to fall for the confirmation bias. That is it looks for things that prove what it already believes to be true. And the dopamine reinforces that as well. So once you start seeing things to be grateful for, your brain starts looking for more things to be grateful for. That's how the virtuous cycle gets created."[4]

In my cancer battle I made a choice to shift my mindset from fear to determination. Even on the tough days when I could easily get down and give up, I reminded myself of the big picture. I counted my blessings. Amazingly, it works and keeps you focused in the right direction. And as you can see from the information shared by Alex Korb, Ph.D., gratitude causes a chemical change in

---

[4] psychologytoday.com, Alex Korb, Ph.D, *The Grateful Brain*, November 20, 2012.

the brain, which then starts a process for the brain to essentially continue down the same path.

I've included a letter my brother wrote before I competed in the IRONMAN World Championship at Kona in 2016, after my cancer surgery. I believe he makes poignant points about mindset and how it keeps you from never giving up.

"Dear Kona,

Next Saturday, you have a rendezvous with my brother Tom Hulsey as well as all the other competitors, at IRONMAN World Championship, the Super Bowl of triathlons. Understand, we all know you will put up a fight, that you will not go quietly into the good night. The conditions you'll throw at them are downright inhumane from rough surf to unforgiving and unrelenting heat to time that never seems to end. You intend to break them, to cause them to lose their will to keep going, and ultimately, to quit.

But understand this, my friend; you don't know Tom and you will find him to be most uncooperative with your plan. To Tom, the word "quit" is the ultimate and unmentionable four-letter word. It is a word that does not exist in his vocabulary, and frankly, he has no time to waste learning what it means. Try as you might, he will not quit.

Instead, you will find Tom to be relentless. He will not stop regardless of conditions, regardless of how he's feeling. This is a man who has stared into the great abyss to overcome cancer in the last year. Sure, he had his down times dealing with it but I never heard him ask why him or feel sorry for himself. Quitting, giving in was never considered. He just kept going and started making new goals. He also realized that he had a message of hope he could spread to others and has done so with ZERO - The End of Prostate Cancer where he has become a valued fundraiser and team member. Just a little over 2 months ago, he competed in the full IRONMAN Lake Placid 2016. You ask did he finish? Of course he did! What kind of question is that?

You need to understand that long before cancer, his outlook on life was formed. In the '60s, Tom grew up in Wisconsin during the glory years of the Green & Gold, listening and learning the gospel of Lombardi. Nothing short of giving it your best and going beyond your abilities wasn't just something that sounded nice – It was expected and anything less was not tolerated. I know this to be completely true as I was lectured many times as Tom's little brother. Later, Tom was further shaped by the 1980 Miracle on Ice. While he loved the team and reveled in the Miracle, he most admired Herb Brooks, the coach responsible for putting the team together. Brooks was another coach who expected nothing but the best and would do everything to ensure the success of the team including some of the best mind games ever. I have no doubt that if Tom had played for Team USA, he would have been the guy wanting to keep skating Brooks' infamous "Herbies" when the rest of the team was dropping. In years since, I've heard Tom say that if he could have, he would have loved to have played for Lombardi and Brooks.

I give you this brief glimpse into the background of Tom Hulsey to let you know that no matter what you throw at Tom on Saturday to stop him, you will fail. If anything, the more obstacles presented during IRONMAN, the more determined and motivated Tom will be. You should move on to the next person because I assure you that you will be disappointed. Your efforts to break Tom will be unsuccessful.

Good luck, Tom! You can and will do it! Expect nothing less than the best and go for it!

Brian Hulsey"

Remember with mindset to always look up and forward to what lies ahead and beyond your current challenge, struggle or goal. The right mindset takes courage and diligence. It can help you step out of your comfort zone. Your mindset drives the choices you make, and the habits you create.

Reflective Questions

Describe your current mindset? Does it need to change? How?

What belief systems hold you back from living your best life?

What steps can you take to improve your mindset?

Persevere

Persevere

"Never give in, never give in, never, never, never, never in nothing great or small, large or petty, never give in except to convictions of honor and sense."

Winston Churchill,

Speech to students at Harrow Hall in 1941

Perseverance figures prominently for any athlete. Even athletes born with incredible, earth-shattering ability and talent must still work hard to perform. Truly, very gifted athletes have something that others don't, but it also takes many years of practice, building skills, pushing through setbacks and sometimes climbing a seemingly too-steep slope to see the payoff.

According to *Outliers* author Malcolm Gladwell, to master a skill to an expert level you must work at it for ten thousand hours. That's 1250 eight-hour days . . . about three-and-a-half-years of practicing and honing a skill every day. I say that to make the point that hard work pays off for anyone who wants to achieve something in life. And hard work takes perseverance. No matter what you are trying to achieve, you might have to fight through something to get to your goal. Even if your desired achievement seems small to others, it belongs to you. Don't let others discourage you.

Perseverance is also a requirement for the actual IRONMAN competition. In spite of what can go wrong in the lengthy race, you have to keep stroking through the water, pumping the bike pedals or pounding the pavement, putting one foot in front of the other. Competing in an IRONMAN requires great tenacity! That tenacity starts months before with the intense mental and physical training, day in and day out. Perseverance keeps the daily training from feeling like drudgery, because it keeps your focus forward, toward the goal, knowing that accomplishing it will provide great satisfaction and fulfillment.

This perseverance as an athlete has been a part of me my whole life and saved my life when I faced cancer. Every day I had to mentally focus on fighting the battle. But I found some days extremely difficult, and I had days when I wanted to give in, but my perseverance kept me going. I don't mean to make it sound easy, I had some really bad days. I had to fight for that perseverance.

Perseverance puts you in a winning rhythm, something I needed for my most challenging race . . . a race for my life against cancer. I never expected to compete in that race. I never planned for it, and that made it much more difficult.

Planning and training for a long-distance race starts many months beforehand with meticulously mapped training for each day. And you have control of it in a sense. Now, instead of planning how far to cycle, swim or run, I had to plan to live. Instead of running away from cancer, I had to learn to face it, to face how it might crimp my lifestyle. Every single day, perseverance helped me take the next step in the walker, work through the pain and believe that I could win the race.

This quote from Dave Scott, six-time IRONMAN world champion about competing at Kona, has inspired me for many years, because it urges me to keep going.

"It's not the distance that overwhelms people who race Hawaii's IRONMAN. It's the relentless wind that blows across the lava fields. You're on the highest ridges, you see miles of repetitive road to Hawaii, and you realize it's extremely hot and you're going straight into 30-mile an hour crosswind. I've found that those who dwell on those conditions tend to fold. I always train for adversity. I always consider adversity an asset, something to turn around to my advantage. One of life's most important lessons is learning to put your losses in perspective and savor your triumphs by riding on euphoria's wave. Have high goals and expectations; regard defeats as strategies on the road to success by remembering the little victories that have gotten you where you are."

Persevere

I've had that quote hanging on my office wall 20 years. It never resonated with me more than over the past three. I've learned that I'm a lot tougher than I thought, and it's actually strengthened me.

Perseverance often separates people who accomplish great things from those who don't. Some people willingly do anything to accomplish their goal. Others fade or give in to discouragement. This applies to something as simple as minor surgery to battling cancer, to everyday life complexities. The mind can overcome almost anything. Perseverance is a tool of the mind to keep on going in spite of the circumstances and what seems reasonably possible.

In the early days of my cancer battle, when I spoke to my friend Jan Klodner who encouraged me to set goals, I found that having something in the future like short-term, intermediate and long-term goals to focus on would help me persevere.

For my short-term goal, I wanted to represent the North Texas Crime Commission on a Mission trip to Seattle 27 days after my surgery. The full agenda included non-stop meetings with organizations such as Microsoft, Amazon and the Port Authority. It wore me down, but I persevered. Lack of strength and bladder control created interesting challenges.

For my intermediate goal, I wanted to complete a half IRONMAN. Exactly six months after surgery I completed the 70.3

Austin IRONMAN with great friends Steve Zuehlke and Willy Waks.

Though not a full IRONMAN, the Austin race represented the most significant goal in my journey back. Medically speaking, it takes 18 months to recover from a Robotic Prostatectomy. So, in Austin I was still early in my recovery, both physically and emotionally (I still didn't talk about my cancer).

The cancer knocked me off my feet, physically, mentally and emotionally undermining all the traits needed to compete in an IRONMAN. I knew it would be a tough road, but I wasn't going to let cancer or the IRONMAN beat me. A half-IRONMAN was a very aggressive goal, but I've always "pushed the envelope" with testing my limits. I had seven abdominal incisions from the surgery and I wondered how my healing core muscles would hold up. I didn't have much time to ramp up training, so I had to play a balancing act between adequate training and not hurting myself because I lost so much of my base fitness in the weeks after surgery.

In the past, when I decided to do a race, my race training built on a foundation of my fitness. Not this time. I literally had to start at ground zero with my overall fitness.

I had so much doubt. Could I even make it through the first leg – the swim? The bike included a lot of hills. Could I climb? If I had to walk during the run that would be okay. I knew I could get to the finish line by putting one foot in front of the other. Could I finish the race? If I finished, my time was irrelevant. I viewed getting to the start line as a victory and celebration of life.

I had such an amazing team supporting me in Austin, an immeasurable asset. Lauren, Steve and Willy gave me so much support. I was challenged in that race, but somehow, I stayed focused and persevered to the finish. Emotions flowed at the finish line. There were lots of hugs and tears of joy. This was a genuine celebration of life!

For my long-term goal, I planned to complete a full IRONMAN in 2016. I signed up for IRONMAN Lake Placid, held 14 months after surgery in July 2016, not knowing if I'd be around to do it. Just in case, for the first time ever, I purchased withdrawal entry fee insurance. I didn't want to risk losing my $800 entry fee.

I created another unexpected goal on Easter 2015, when Matthew Palmore asked for permission to marry my daughter Michelle. He proposed to her and they set their wedding date for July 2016, just three weeks before IRONMAN Lake Placid. All of a sudden I had very tangible and urgent reasons to not give up, to persevere. Two long-term goals drove me to never, never give up. July 2016, a memorable month, brought with it two life-defining moments.

Lake Placid, 2016

Lake Placid race day, 2016 challenged my belief in myself, and my ability to totally overcome cancer and its drain on me. This goes back to perseverance. The mishaps and challenges on that day just made me a stronger person, a better fighter. As I said earlier, perseverance just drives you to the win. In my case, winning meant finishing the race.

The 2.4-mile swim was brutal. There were almost 3,000 athletes competing . . . that's 12,000 churning limbs. Who said swimming is not a contact sport? Imagine being in a washing machine or playing hockey without pads. That's what a triathlon swim is like.

I injured my shoulder in a skiing accident just four months before this race. When hit or hitting others during the swim stroke, pain seared through me, but I pushed forward. Receiving a hit or hitting others during the swim stroke was painful. This does not happen when you train in a pool with a lane to yourself. You can't avoid contact in this situation, but it definitely hurts and saps energy.

IRONMAN swim strategy dictates that you save your energy for the long day ahead. When I competed in that race I still had challenges as I recovered from surgery. Getting kicked in the face and getting a bloody nose in this race was not a good way to start the day!

The 112-mile bike assaulted my recovering sore shoulder. All the vibration of the bike ride transfers to the shoulders. I had to change three flat tires, which did not help my time. Also, since one of the side effects from my surgery was bladder control, I had to stop at every aid station, every 10 miles – yikes! Hotter weather would have helped, since sweating means fewer visits to the port-a-potty. Unfortunately for me, we had mild race day temperatures. By most standards it was beautiful and pleasant, but not for a guy who needed to sweat to stay away from port-a-potties. Those stops robbed me of precious minutes.

The 26.2-mile run started out well. My shoulder felt better. The discomfort shifted to my feet. I developed hot spots, eventually covering a majority of the bottom of both feet, making each strike to the ground painful. I stopped to get medical aid and they recommended soaking my feet in ice water. I reluctantly agreed, knowing this would take precious time. The ice worked . . . for about 10 miles, then, the pain came back, so I returned to the medical tent for the same treatment (in total, almost a half hour). With the focus on my feet, I neglected nutrition and grew weak and dizzy. Even though I never drink cola, I had some at the last aid station. It gave me some quick energy that helped sustain me to the finish line.

I got to the finish line at this IRONMAN, but I fought the whole way, both physically and mentally. I had completed every race I started and I was determined that this race would not be my first DNF (did not finish).

During those really tough times in the darkness on the run at Lake Placid, I kept thinking about the reasons I chose this race. I set it as a goal to help me focus beyond my health issues. I meant to honor my friend Bill Rollings, who succumbed to prostate cancer way too young, and, to inspire others. I staggered to the finish with less than 22 minutes to spare, at 11:39 p.m.! What a long day!

Steve Zuehlke supported me through my entire journey. He finished ahead of me on this day and I found him waiting at the finish line for me with his wife Sue, and Lauren. I hadn't seen him since before the swim start. Despite being physically and mentally drained, the finish line was an amazing experience to share with them!

Perseverance – Life Skill

"It's not whether you get knocked down; it's whether you get up."

This quote by my idol, Coach Vince Lombardi has served as one of my mantras throughout life, and it never resonated more with me than at IRONMAN Lake Placid.

I crossed the finish line at Lake Placid, but as you can see, it did not come without challenges. Everything that could go wrong went wrong. Getting to the finish line of this race required mental strength like no other. I barely made the 17-hour cut-off at midnight. That rattled me to the core, to the point where I wondered if going to Kona and competing at the IRONMAN World Championship eleven weeks later was feasible. Doubt and fear crept in. Maybe cancer had taken more out of me than I realized.

The Support System

Perseverance comes from within, but a loving and positively minded support system fortifies it. Completing IRONMAN Lake Placid 2016 was the long-term goal that I set for 17 months after my diagnosis. Lake Placid is considered one of the toughest IRONMAN courses in the world due to the elevation changes.

Many asked, "Why didn't you choose an easier one?"

My answer, "I wouldn't have it any other way!"

Honestly, I needed a lofty goal to pull me out of the ditch and the mental downward spiral instigated by my cancer diagnosis. And, the goal took perseverance that my support system truly fortified.

My wife Lauren's unflinching support over those months, kept me going and focusing on my long-term goal. I had someone constantly encouraging and believing in me and helping me believe I could do it. When doubt or concern crept in, she reminded me of why I picked the tough goal and that I had to stick with it the way I have all my life.

Another great friend in my life is fellow health club member Todd Carter. Todd always provides encouragement. His upbeat personality turns me to the positive outcome. Friends like Todd are a valuable part of my support system. He helped me stick with a goal, especially a huge and challenging one. When I doubted whether my story could help people, he said,

"Perseverance! This is a trait that many people want but have a hard time accomplishing or getting. This goes for everything in life . . . Your story can motivate people greatly. One man who overcame cancer, beat it down, and still ran an IRONMAN . . . what . . . amazing, how unbelievable! How did you do it? That is your story . . . you did not let anything deter you."

Perseverance does come from within, yet we all need others to help us through life's journey, especially when we have a mountain of a goal to accomplish.

How Can Perseverance Help You?

Ask yourself, what do you face in your life right now that requires perseverance? What challenge do you have, no matter how small, that tenacity could help you journey through? Your challenge may not be cancer, but we all have life challenges. Maybe you have something going on that you feel is out of your control. Know that, despite what you may think, you can take action, to get through it. If you need to, ask for help from friends, family or professionals. I had friends to help me get in the right mindset and medical professionals to guide me through treatment options.

Take the first step and set goals like I did to get through cancer. When you do this, even in the most discouraging times, the goals will give you something to focus on, to move toward. When your situation looks bleak remember that it is only temporary. You have to keep moving forward one step at a time no matter what.

You must consistently proclaim and visualize what you want to achieve as though it were reality. Then, when you feel like giving up, train your mind to go to what you have visualized. Perseverance grows into a habit and it comes in handy when you have setbacks, when you feel like you just can't go on.

I have relied on that perseverance during my life; it's one of the things that gave me the courage and ability to fight the daily battle with cancer. When you stare death squarely in the face, you must embrace that daily challenge to keep pushing forward, to keep believing and doing what you need to do to live.

And, at times, I truly felt ready to give up. But I kept my focus, and mental drive to look beyond what stood right in front of me. You can do the same. Even if you find it easier to give up, you can change that at any point in your life. You can choose to persevere. Sometimes, you just have to take the first step and say to yourself, "I always persevere, in spite of what happens, in spite of all obstacles."

Perseverance means keeping on with something even when you don't see immediate results. It comes from having the faith and tenacity to know that the process will produce the results.

As you can see from my story, it helps to have a support group around you to persevere through the curve balls that life throws at you. If you don't have one, find one, make one, form one.

Sometimes that takes courage. Maybe you're single and live away from family. Find people who will support you through life. This often starts with giving to others. You will reap what you sow. Giving support to others will always come back to you in one form or another.

Keep going and remember what Vince Lombardi said,

"It's not whether you get knocked down; it's whether you get up."

Reflective Questions

"It's not whether you get knocked down; it's whether you get up."

— Vince Lombardi

How does this quote apply to your life? Can you remember a time when you got knocked down and you got up? What did you gain from it?

If you feel like you've been knocked down and can't get up, who can you call on or what can do?

When you do recover from the fall, how will your life change for the better?

Be Intentional

"When you get right down to it, intentional living is about living your best story."

John C. Maxwell

Being intentional has proven easier for me post-cancer, for two reasons. One, I had very specific goals to get through my cancer fight and, two, I was competing for something greater than myself; a cause that could make a positive impact on society. Today, I find motivation to be intentional by knowing that I can provide hope and inspiration to cancer patients. I lead exercise classes at the Baylor, Scott & White Cancer Health & Wellness Center, to help patients through recovery and beyond. I love to see the expression in their eyes that says, "If he can do it, I can, too!"

As a result, my conviction to help other cancer patients added to being intentional in my life.

Maintaining a winning mindset comes from a conscious choice. As I mentioned earlier, a key component of a winning mindset is being intentional. As an adult, I have typically done so with my health and life. I'll admit, it hasn't been easy and I'm not perfect. It takes focus and attention to what I eat, how I exercise, how I operate in the business world, in personal relationships and working toward a goal.

Living intentionally for me has always included nutrition. I use the analogy of the automobile engine. If you put junk in the gas tank, the car won't perform well. So, I don't eat fried foods, sugary desserts or white flour – most of the time! Truly, "You are what you eat."

I stopped competing in endurance events in 1993 to focus on my children. Though I continued to eat the "right" foods and set an example for my kids, I didn't reduce my caloric intake based on my body's needs. Because I had stopped competing in endurance events, I didn't need the same amount of calories for fuel.

The weight loss and control industry is a billion dollar business, and yet you can maintain the right weight with a very simple equation. Caloric intake should equal calories burned. My intake exceeded calories burned. As a result, my weight ballooned from 175 to over 200 pounds. Until this point in my life, weight had never been a concern for me with the high volume of training I did.

Even though I maintained high physical activity, since I was on the ice several times a week as a hockey coach and instructor and at the gym daily, my training regimen was not the same since I was not training for endurance events. I simply wasn't burning as many calories.

I fell into the trap of rationalizing that I was eating healthy food and I would start eating less tomorrow. The saying "You are what you eat" had a new meaning to me. I had to buy new pants to fit my expanding waistline and shirts that fit my new collar size.

A defining moment in this season in my life came when my young daughter, Michelle teased me by saying, "Dad, look at that gut."

Oh, the brutal honesty of kids. She clearly sounded the wakeup call I needed. She embarrassed me into a challenge, and I took it.

At that time, in my 40s, I knew I needed more discipline in my eating. Eating too much food, whether nutritious or not, is not healthy. I recognized that I had chosen a wrong path toward high blood pressure, obesity and high cholesterol. I was accidentally overweight because I failed to be intentional about what and how much I ate compared to the calories that I burned.

I love margaritas, but they are fattening! One night in 2005, during dinner, Lauren asked me if there were one thing I wanted to do in my life, what would it be. I told her I that I wanted to compete in the IRONMAN again. When Lauren gave me her blessing to compete again, I made a conscious decision not to drink alcohol. I did not drink alcohol from that night until after I completed the

World Championship in 2016. I made that commitment to myself and Lauren, and maintained my conscious choice. Of course I had days when drinking a margarita sounded good, but I had to continually make the choice not to drink one. It's just about being conscious and intentional.

Accidentally Overweight

As I mentioned earlier, I got careless with how much I ate and gained about 25 pounds, almost by accident. Libby Weaver, MD has written a book, *Accidentally Overweight,* which provides guidance for a healthy diet. She describes how gaining weight can creep up on us. She says, regarding how much we eat, "You know you cannot eat like a piglet and expect everything to fall into place. That's just common sense." [5]

She describes how many times we leave work late, stressed out, so we grab some fast food on the way home and chill out, stretched out on the couch. Then, we do it all over again the next day. We just need to make the right daily choices.

Eating fast food one time won't kill you, but over time that same choice will make a huge difference in your health.

She also talks about how stress impacts your digestive system and health. Adrenaline, intended to help you stand and fight or get you out of danger fast, promotes the "fight or flight" response

---

[5] *Accidentally Overweight*, Dr. Libby Weaver

by sending blood to your extremities for added strength and speed. Adrenalin causes a sugar dump to the bloodstream, which in turn prompts insulin to curb the sugar spike. Insulin also serves as the fat-storing hormone. This chain reaction served us well thousands of years ago, but in modern times, you may experience stress while sitting at your desk, driving to the office or talking to a difficult client or colleague. You don't burn the sugar to get out of danger. Any sugar that your body doesn't burn gets stored as fat. Over time those stressful days can add to your waistline.

Without getting into too much detail, Cortisol is our long-term stress hormone, For example, at one point it protected people from scarcity of food. It can signal your body about the lack of food, so it slows down your metabolism to preserve the fuel supply. Again, the stress that creates this response in modern time, in most cases is not life threatening, but the impact on the chemical makeup of your body is the same. You don't need the hormone to save you from starving because we have plenty of food, and, if you don't exert more physical activity than normal, this can potentially cause weight-gain and contribute to metabolic syndrome. Metabolic syndrome is a condition of elevated blood pressure, elevated cholesterol and insulin resistance. Insulin resistance can warn of potential Type II Diabetes.

Stress you need to avoid obviously depends on your situation. You can choose not to be stressed, when you learn different ways to react to situations, or choose to change your environment. The same goes for choosing the right food, exercising, getting enough sleep and drinking the right amount of water. In my life I have found that those small daily intentional choices totally impact my life whether I'm training for a triathlon, fighting cancer or helping companies dispel cyber attacks.

In hindsight, I needed definitive goals to keep me intentional about my weight. When I had goals for competing in triathlons, I maintained focus on the right weight for me, because weight is so integrated into the success of the race. When I wasn't preparing for those races, I stopped paying close attention to what I consumed. If I had tracked my eating habits, I would have had a much easier time figuring out how to cut back.

Intentional Healthy Lifestyle

"In a world that profits from chronic disease, taking care of your body is a rebellious act." – Author unknown

Just as gaining weight resulted from my choice because I wasn't paying close attention and making excuses for how much I ate, you have to choose a healthy lifestyle. This doesn't have to be a daunting undertaking, if you make realistic changes without letting yourself off the hook. For example, maybe you know you need to stop drinking so much caffeine. You could start by drinking a 50/50 mix of caffeinated and non-caffeinated coffee, with a specific date when you will stop drinking caffeine all together. As another example, perhaps you don't eat enough fruits and vegetables. Make it a habit to eat 5-7 servings of fruits and vegetables a day, and track it on your phone. Find fruits and veggies that you really like. You'll be amazed at how full you'll feel.

To keep yourself motivated, remember the benefits of the healthy lifestyle. Long- term, eating a balanced diet, getting regular exercise and maintaining a healthy weight can add years to your life. Poor lifestyle choices, such as smoking, overuse of alcohol, poor diet, lack of physical activity and inadequate relief of chronic stress are key contributors in the development and progression of preventable chronic diseases.

You have to choose a healthy lifestyle, just like choosing to sit in front of the television for an average of five hours per day[6] as many Americans do. Can you say, "couch potato"? My Dad called the television the idiot box. Watching mindless hours of television has all the benefits of eating junk foods. In a 65-year life, that person will have spent nine years glued to the tube.

Make a Commitment

In our society, a healthy lifestyle requires commitment. The majority of American adults are overweight or obese, and weight is a growing problem among US children. According to Institute for Health Metrics & Evaluation, "the highest proportion of overweight

---

[6] "Cross-Platform Report", Nielsen Media Ratings Company

and obese people – 13 percent of the global total – live in the United States, a country which accounts for only 5 percent of the world's population. An estimated 160 million Americans are either obese or overweight. Nearly three-quarters of American men and more than 60% of women are obese or overweight." [7]

Fact: one can of soda contains 10 teaspoons of sugar and the average American adult drinks 500 cans of soda every year, estimating about 52 pounds of sugar consumed in soft drinks alone. The longer you follow healthy behaviors, the easier you find it to continue them, and best of all, you actually start to enjoy them.

The first step for adopting a healthy lifestyle is attitude. It takes time and perseverance, but your body will adapt. For example, the way your body feels after a healthy meal will become more important to you than the instant pleasure of having something loaded with fat or sugar. Not only will your body change, but your mind will change as well. These changes come over time, sometimes weeks, months or years of slowly working on your habits and choices. Allow yourself this crucial time for permanent change.

If you keep giving your best effort, your quality of life will improve. Sometimes you won't see changes overnight, and for that reason many people give up before they see the results of the changes. Old habits die hard. Take it one day at a time, one healthy

---

[7] Institute for Health Metrics & Evaluation

choice at a time. Just like when I ran in the IRONMANs, I kept putting one foot in front of the other and taking it one step at a time. If I hadn't done that, the goal of finishing might have seemed too daunting. Use the same logic as I used when setting goals in my recovery from cancer . . . one step at a time.

Small Right Choices

In his book *The Slight Edge* Jeff Olson talks about the idea of making right daily choices. He describes how a brilliant athlete didn't just walk on the court or the field one day and start performing amazing feats. The amazing performance came from hours and hours, and years and years of hard work, out of the public eye. That athlete made right daily choices that added up to the skill, abilities and performance that we see today.

Deciding not to do a workout today, or skipping part of it, won't put you totally out of shape, but if you continue to make that small wrong choice it will grow into a habit that impacts you negatively. Drinking the right amount of water today won't instantly make you healthy, but drinking the right amount of water daily can have positive impact on your skin and brain function. Watching your favorite mindless TV shows for a couple of hours tonight won't make you a couch potato unless you continue to do it night after night. You could make a better choice by reading or taking a walk every night, even if only for 30 minutes. The first few nights, you might find it hard to make the change, but over time reading or taking that walk becomes the new habitual behavior. These small choices make you intentional about your health.

The healthy choices definitely have a positive impact. For one, you'll have more energy and focus. If you look at highly successful people, like Warren Buffet for example, who spends a fair amount of time reading, they have healthy habits. Most likely, when they discover themselves falling into a bad habit they stop and make a change. Tony Robbins has a routine he follows every morning to get going and to ensure that he has the energy to motivate thousands of people across the globe. He makes the right choice every morning to follow that ritual.

Your mindset plays into a healthy lifestyle too. If you find yourself angry a lot of the time, find out why and learn to deal with life in a different way. Negative emotions wreak havoc on your health. And when you have healthy emotions, you'll have better all-round quality of life and enjoyment.

Healthy choices may require some change for you that you don't like, but in the long-term the change will benefit you. Intentionally take one day at a time. Make one good choice at a time.

Pay Attention!

Being intentional also means to pay attention! How many times do we drive somewhere and realize when we get there, that we operated essentially on autopilot? Our brains are wired to follow habitual patterns, so sometimes we have to fight our brain to take intentional action that might be different than our typical pattern.

My mom taught me that pain is the body's way of warning you of something wrong. Don't ignore it. Listen! Diligently listening to your body is part of being intentional about your health. If you have pain, figure out why. I've never embraced taking painkillers as they mask the pain, risking possible further injury. And they all have side effects. Even the "wonder drug" aspirin, has side effects by affecting the stomach lining.

Recently, I experienced pain in my upper left chest. Initially, I thought it was a by-product of my recent rotator cuff surgery. I ignored it at first, because I had no other symptoms, but the pain persisted. My mom's voice, in my head, reminded me of what she had always taught me. So, I figured I should get it checked out by a cardiologist. The EKG came back fine. The cardiologist agreed that it probably had something to do with the shoulder. We then decided that as a precaution, I should take a stress test. As a cardio junkie, I had no worries. No way I could have an issue with blockage. Bring it!

The stress test changed everything. It showed 90 percent blockage in one of the arteries. Again, a diagnosis knocked the wind out of me. A stream of questions and worries streamed through my head. Why me? What did I do wrong? I thought my commitment to cardio would have prevented any issues with blockage. I survived cancer, now this? Again, the thoughts of what would happen to me came flooding back. How would this impact my life long-term?

The doctor insisted I have the stents put in immediately. Panic set in. My wife immediately flew home from her business trip. Two stents later, all is good. Be intentional with your health and the signals your body gives you. If I had not been paying attention, I might not be here.

Intentional Game Plan

After getting over the shock, denial, and anger of learning I had cancer, which took about a month, Lauren and I developed a game plan. I accepted the fact that I was staring down the biggest challenge of my life. I committed a lot of time to conducting due-diligence on the options for fighting prostate cancer. I researched and interviewed specialists regarding the different treatment options. I committed to being in the best shape possible in order to give my body the best chance of a quicker recovery. I trained like I was getting ready for an IRONMAN. I wanted to take advantage and leverage my fitness. Setting goals was the best thing I did in anticipation of my post-surgery recovery. Though not new for me, this strategy prepared me for the biggest challenge in my life. Goals created structure for my game plan and helped me to act intentionally, and this was key both physically and mentally.

Specific goals set you on a path that you choose. Goals, when you stick to them, make you accountable for taking intentional actions. You can ask yourself if your actions have taken you closer to, or further away from your goal.

An Intentional Life

One of the life lessons I always want to teach young people is "be intentional in your life," especially in your 20s and 30s. This is the foundation for the rest of your life. The decisions you make daily during this period, good and bad, will carry forward the rest of your life, especially decisions regarding health. I've always strived to be a role model and to walk the talk, for my own kids and students. As a hockey coach and instructor, I've tried to be a positive influence on children, both on and off the ice.

As one mother wrote, "You are a giant as a mentor, an athlete, an artist, and a role model. Hundreds of children benefitted from your knowledge, experience, and especially your happy, positive demeanor. Our community is fortunate to claim you!"

Such comments humble and elate me. To know that I truly impacted someone's life gives me a wonderful feeling, and, a great responsibility. I believe that the reason that I have successfully impacted others starts with being intentional about who I am and what I do.

I've worked with children from many less-than-ideal backgrounds, including those with drug addiction and abusive parents. Connecting with people and meeting their needs has always been one of my strengths. Fortunately, God has shown me the way to use those gifts to help others. With many kids, it started with a common interest in hockey and skating and an almost immediate bond. Circumstances forced us to spend a lot of time together. Many saw me as a father figure. I even went to court for one of my students in a custody battle. As a good listener, intentionally lending an empathetic ear, I was always able to build strong relationships with my students. My hockey mantra, "Keep your stick low and goals high," resonated with many of my students. After rocky starts, many of my students have gone on to live successful lives. I like to believe that getting really clear about their daily choices and actions enabled them to do well in life.

Even in my dealings with my students I set goals. I influenced these children and added value to their families because I modeled and taught them self-discipline, teamwork and perseverance. These are the tools they needed to be intentional in their lives. Being intentional about everything from what you say to what you do helps you take charge of your life, rather than letting it take charge of you.

Here's a something Danya Nardozza, a parent of two of my students said.

"You have always exuded positivity, generosity and warmth. These are the reasons we returned to you for lessons. Not just fantastic skill building, but so that my son and daughter could witness and be in the presence of a true athlete. A man of honor and integrity, self-discipline, teamwork and perseverance were the life skills gained from healthy pursuits, and these would be the real gifts of skating. Meeting you was one of the best things that have happened to my children—our family!"

I love to hear about the impact I had on someone's life by being intentional in my coaching methods, yet, the student always makes the choice.

Staying Focused

Being intentional will keep you focused. If you start a new business or other venture, you have to focus on your goal. You have to be intentional about your everyday actions. That intention with your actions will keep you focused.

At Kona in the swim, competitors have to deal with the mighty swells of the Pacific Ocean. Think of all the power in that body of water. It takes additional focus to stay on track in that swim. To swim most efficiently you have to navigate a straight line, as much as possible, toward the next buoy, because the swells can easily throw you off track.

I remember having to constantly focus on the buoy and adjust, with the concern of losing time and energy in the swim due to fighting the ocean's current. This increases the challenge, because in an IRONMAN you compete against time and your body's stamina. You don't want to waste any energy on swimming out of line. You must complete the swim and get out of the water as quickly as possible.

I find this so similar to the events and things we deal with in life. Perhaps you work in a chaotic corporate environment where competing agendas pull you in different directions. Sometimes it requires you to stop and re-prioritize your work. Perhaps you have competing priorities in your life. Your employer wants you to be on call whenever they need you; your family needs your support and attention; the non-profit you volunteer for really appreciates your time, so you give it freely; and your friends need your attention. In this situation you need to intentionally guard your time. This can mean some hard choices. Some people will steal your time when you need to guard it. Some will get offended if you are not there when they need you.

You have to be honest with people about what you can and can't reasonably do. Spend your time intentionally, even if you have lots of priorities pulling at you. Managing multiple priorities is truly like swimming in the swells of the ocean. Those priorities can easily pull you off track. Sometimes you may have to focus on one thing at a time. When you are at home, focus on your family. When at work, focus on the work, and learn to say no to some activities and obligations.

Being Intentional Even When You Don't Feel Like It

As an early riser, I do most of my workouts early in the morning. It takes discipline and focus to get up at 4:30 on a cold morning. Some days, I just may not feel like it, but I know I have to do it to prepare for an endurance event, and, to prepare for life. Focusing on the results I'm looking for helps me forge through if I don't feel like it.

I just think of my reward, knowing how I will feel after the workout and shower; like a million bucks and ready to take on the world. Some people get up early and read or meditate. Whatever your motivation, be intentional! I always know those early morning workouts created the strong foundation for my overall fitness as I prepared for that big goal – IRONMAN!

Intention in Various Facets of Life

You can be intentional in all facets of your life, both personal and professional. My career passion of making the world a safer place by leveraging technology means I have to keep abreast of a rapidly changing technology landscape. That is not an easy task. Being intentional about my focus, has always led me to understand what any technology actually provides the organization. As a cyber-security consultant, I leveraged my ability to relate with senior leaders in order to serve as a critical resource. I used my abilities to protect an organization's data, including trade secrets and customer information to serve that passion of making the world a safer place.

Where can you be more intentional in your life? How will that impact you and those around you? Examining these questions could start you on the path to changing habitual negative patterns in your life. Being intentional can move you toward your goals and dreams because you pay closer attention. Be intentional and improve your life!

Karen Salmansohn, founder of NotSalmon.com, sums it up well.

"If you want to improve your life you must commit to changing your daily habits and creating permanent lifestyle shift. You can't depend on quick fixes."

Reflective Questions

Where could you be more intentional in your life?

How will that help you through life's daily challenges?

How can you be intentional about helping others?

Overcome Your Fear

Overcome Your Fear

"If you want to conquer fear, don't sit home and think about it. Go out and get busy."

Dale Carnegie

When I heard my urologist say those three words, "You have cancer;" fear and disbelief overwhelmed me. Until that fateful day I thought of myself as an IRONMAN— invincible. Suddenly, that view of myself was shattered. Fear overwhelmed me. Fear entered my thoughts every day and began to overtake my vision for the rest of my life. Between each doctor visit the questions rolled around in my head.

Was I going to be one of those men who dies every 19 minutes from prostate cancer? Would I experience a long, painful decline like my friend Bill Rollings? What is going to happen to me? What will my battle with cancer be like? Is it even worth fighting?

I was paralyzed.

I did not want to talk about it and that compounded my situation. Keeping it to myself allowed the fear to grow stronger like the idea of false evidence that appears real. When you don't talk about it or process it, it just gets bigger. In addition, I had never had to deal with fear of this magnitude before.

After my first elevated PSA reading, the doctor told me not to worry. An infection could cause the spike. Easier said than done. I had to return in six months, then three months and then again in six months to get my PSA checked. My PSA kept rising, so between each visit I had all the angst about what my next test would reveal. I knew this would not end well. I had a sense of hopelessness, especially with the memory of Bill's battle.

Bill was diagnosed with metastatic castration resistant prostate cancer. This particular cancer grows while on androgen deprivation therapy (ADT) and spreads to the bones, organs and lymph nodes. Initially he had a radical prostatectomy, followed by salvage radiation along with Lupron. Over the next four years, he underwent other therapies and clinical trials. The last trial consisted of Radium 223 infusions at Tulane University. Eventually, they told him they could do nothing more. Having witnessed Bill lose his gut-wrenching battle with prostate cancer, just months before my

PSA spiked, I just about gave up. I did not want to go through what Bill went through.

I feared what people would think. I had been almost arrogant about my health. I was so overcome with fear that I decided I couldn't talk to anyone about having cancer. Only two people knew about my diagnosis.

I had all but decided to let the cancer run its course rather than go through the battle my friend suffered. My fear took over. I did not want to lose my masculinity, wear a diaper and have to use a walker. All treatments have quality-of-life side effects. I did not want to have to deal with them. Fear devastated my mindset and led me down a mental path so different from my nature.

Fighting the Fear and the Cancer

Thank goodness for Lauren's encouragement. She reminded me that I am a fighter, and, she wanted me around for the long haul. We both knew this would be a tough battle, where we were literally fighting for my life. I say we were fighting the battle because with her encouragement, I decided to a least look at treatment options. About this same time I had that attitude-changing conversation with Jan Klodner.

In my challenge to overcome my fear, I thought about something author Maria Coffey said,

"The hardest, most challenging experiences of our lives can enrich our existence, revealing our true identity, awakening us to greater awareness of our own potential, and opening us to the infinite beauty of the universe."

This quote really resonates with me because I found dealing with cancer a great physical and mental challenge. I always enjoyed perfect health and I was pro-active about it, so I didn't understand how this happened to me. Overcoming my fear eventually led me to get past the fact that I had cancer and subsequently to figure out how to help others who faced the same situation.

As Maria Coffey said, this struggle with cancer and my fear actually made me a stronger person and led me to a calling to help others facing the same battle. I know that the support of friends and loved ones got me through, so I want to lend a helping hand to others. It gives me great joy to give people hope for the future and encouragement to beat cancer or whatever challenge they have in life.

Acknowledge the Fear without Focus

To overcome fear, you must acknowledge it, yet not focus on it. Naysayers can feed your fear and chip away at your belief. So, in addition to keeping your own head clear of fear, you have to surround yourself with people who don't focus on fear. You may find it difficult to totally escape some of the naysayers because they exist among your co-workers, or family members that you talk with on a regular basis. You have to set up boundaries to protect yourself. You have to surround yourself with like-minded people who have a positive outlook on life.

Teddy Roosevelt said

"It is not the critic who counts; not the man who points out how the strong man stumbled or where the doer of deeds could have done them better. The credit belongs to the man who is actually in the arena, whose face is marred by dust and sweat and blood; who strives valiantly; who errs and comes short again and again; who knows great enthusiasms, the great devotions; who spends himself in a worthy cause; who at the best, knows in the end the triumph of high achievement, and who, at the worst, if he fails, at least fails while daring greatly so that his place shall never be with those timid souls who neither know victory nor defeat."

This quote inspired me to enter my first IRONMAN in 1986. I had it posted on the mirror in the bathroom as a constant reminder of what I wanted to achieve as I trained for the event.

Fear of a Different Kind

Overcoming my initial fear was key in my battle with cancer and it's interesting how at the same time I was dealing with my cancer battle, a wonderful event, my daughter's wedding was causing great fear too! These were fears I had to get over to play my part in my daughter's special day.

I will always remember that huge moment when I walked my daughter, Michelle, down the aisle in July 2016. I was so proud. Being the father of the bride consisted of more than just walking her down the aisle. Two of my responsibilities required me to overcome and manage two of my biggest fears of public speaking and dancing in front of an audience. Both of these required me to go way outside of my comfort zone. The thought terrified me, but I managed my fears with a lot of practice and support from Lauren and Michelle.

Lauren, a public speaker, assisted me in writing a creative speech, something heartfelt and peppered with humor. We spent countless hours rehearsing. I could not have been more prepared. The more I practiced, the less fear I had. The practice built my confidence and focused my mind in the right direction.

I also had to overcome my fear of dancing. As Lauren pointed out, Michelle has danced all her life and for me to do this would be so endearing. Michelle practiced with me diligently for six weeks, which we kept secret in our own little family circle. Since I have no rhythm, Michelle had to keep a positive can-do attitude. I drew strength to overcome my fear challenges by focusing on how important this was to Michelle. We started with Heartland's "I Loved Her First," then we broke out to Justin Timberlake's "Can't Stop the Feeling." The guests went nuts.

My initial fears about father-of-the-bride duties might have knocked me back temporarily, but I did not let them take over. Making Michelle's special day shine took priority over my fears.

Before the wedding, Michelle wrote me a letter. In part it said, "I am so proud of you for multiple reasons, you are the strongest man I know. Not only physically, but for putting your fears aside for me on my wedding day. It means the world to me."

Attitude Adjustment

Attitude, whether positive or negative counts for everything in life. Overcoming my fear helped me turn the corner to embrace my typical positive attitude. As Coach Lombardi said, life will knock you down. Unfortunate events will happen. How you choose to deal with it impacts your quality of life. What counts is whether you get up when you get knocked down.

After my surgery, it would have been easy to lie around and feel sorry for myself. I had so much pain. I chose to take Coach Lombardi's advice to get up. I chose to have a positive attitude, to focus and visualize beyond my current state. That's where the goals that my friend Jan suggested came in. That focus helped me look forward to a time of good health.

Overcoming my fear led to putting myself back in a positive frame of mind, which is absolutely necessary to train and compete in an IRONMAN and to enjoy the best in life. What you focus on truly shapes you and how you experience life.

As I mentioned, to deal with fear, first you must acknowledge it. Ignoring it won't make it go away. As with any challenges in life, whether it's your health, a tennis match, or competing in an endurance event, start by acknowledging the fear so you can overcome it. If you don't, it will paralyze you.

Overcome Your Fear

Unfortunately, most people cling to their fears. I did for a long time. Learning to deal with fear means putting your negative thoughts in perspective. We tend to focus too much on the negative, so by looking at all the options, I realized that I could respond differently to my concerns.

Instead of thinking of something bad that can happen, think of a positive outcome. Articulate the positive outcome to your fear. For me, my positive outcome meant beating cancer and walking my daughter down the aisle. In the weeks leading up to the World Championship in Hawaii in 2016, I felt fearful and intimidated, especially coming on the heels of my struggles at Lake Placid. I continuously had to flip it by visualizing crossing the finish line. If I had not turned the fear into a vision of success, I doubt I could have accomplished my goals.

What Fears Hold You Back?

What fears hold you back right now? Look at your fears realistically and think about how logical they are. Facing your fears takes courage, but it's the only way to overtake them.

Fear is interesting, especially if you are naturally a worrier. It can create a reality in your mind that has no basis in fact, yet it consumes you. Perception is reality in the eye of the beholder. As a business professional, I've seen fear actually keep people from doing their best work because the worry and concern takes focus from the work or task at hand. In the corporate world, even when a person less skilled attacked someone, the fear could prove overwhelming for the person who was attacked. Fear caused them to overthink their actions, lose sleep at night and actually change their image of the value they brought to the organization.

Designed to protect us from danger, we experience fear as part of the fight or flight response. Marilyn Mitchell, MD, a contributor to psychologytoday.com, says,

> "The fight or flight stress response occurs naturally when we perceive that we are under excessive pressure, and it is designed to protect us from bodily harm. Our sympathetic nervous system becomes immediately engaged in creating a number of physiological changes, including increased metabolism, blood pressure, heart and breathing rate, dilation of pupils, constriction of our blood vessels, all that work to

enable us to fight or flee from a stressful or dangerous situation."[8]

While fear is intended to keep us out of trouble, it can lead to serious health consequences when unfounded. In his book *The Psychology of Winning*, Dr. Denis Waitley[9] refers to a speech given by Dr. Herbert Benson, professor, author, cardiologist, and founder of Harvard's Mind/Body Medical Institute, where Benson describes the power of negative belief in Voodoo practice. In Voodoo ancestor worship, the witch doctor spins a chicken bone in a group of people and the one the bone points to dies of a fear-induced heart attack. The belief that the people have in the witch doctor's ability to curse someone to death, actually causes the person to inflict death on himself.

Dr. Benson coined the term "Relaxation Response," as your personal ability to encourage your body to release chemicals and brain signals that make your muscles and organs slow down and increase blood flow to the brain. In his book, *The Relaxation Response*, Dr. Benson describes the scientific benefits of relaxation, explaining that regular practice of the Relaxation Response can offer an effective treatment for a wide range of stress-related disorders.

---

[8] psychologytoday.com, Marilyn Mitchell, MD, March 29, 2013
[9] *The Psychology of Winning*, Dr. Denis Waitley,

So, when fear holds you back from achieving your dreams and goals, certain techniques like meditation can help your brain get out of it. When fear causes you to feel defeated before you even start a battle, try to overcome a challenge or try doing something you've never done before. Defeat the fear before it defeats you.

If I had not overtaken my fear of defeat by cancer and losing my life, I would not have written this book. Whatever your fear, look at it and see if that emotion is protecting you or destroying you. To succeed, you must put yourself in the right frame of mind to achieve your dreams, overcome obstacles and live your best life.

Reflective Questions

What fears do you have?

How do those fears impact your life?

What can you do today to start overcoming your fear?

Be Prepared

"By failing to prepare, you are preparing to fail."

— Benjamin Franklin

You can handle anything in life if you are prepared. Sometimes our tough trials prepare us for the toughest trials. Being intentional and prepared for an active and healthy life, saved my life in the end.

For me, cancer surgery was a game-changer. I felt like an 18-wheeler ran over me. I was severely challenged, but was mentally prepared.

Once we made the decision to move forward with a radical prostatectomy, I trained physically and mentally as though getting ready for an IRONMAN. I wanted to be in top shape, in hopes of making recovery easier and shorter. The enormity of this challenge came into reality during my pre-operation appointment ten days before surgery.

When I exchanged pleasantries with the nurse, I asked, "How are you?" and she responded, "Better than you."

At that point, my mental toughness took a hit, as evidenced by my blood pressure sky rocketing to 210/100. Yikes! Talk about a curveball. I'm glad I had worked on my own plan to survive the surgery and recover, which helped me calm down.

The anticipation of surgery stressed me on a level similar to the pre-race jitters of a triathlon swim. The swim is intimidating because of the contact nature of the sport. You must prepare yourself mentally and push aside fears of the open water. Murky water adds to the uncertainty because you can't see the thrashing arms and legs, and other things in the water. Add in water currents and swells, and it is not for the faint of heart. Essentially you face many unknowns in the swim. My surgery had a lot of unknowns too. I knew I faced challenges in recovery, yet I knew that I had never experienced a situation where I could not run, swim and bike at will. My physical situation post-surgery was entirely different than anything I had ever experienced in my life.

As with anything in life, the difference between successful people and less successful people depends on how they deal with adversity. Life presents us with lots of challenges and how we choose to deal with them is what separates winners and losers. Mental focus is paramount, and that has to start before you race in a big event or face a big event in your life. You have to prepare with a habit of mental focus. You can't just conjure it up on race day. Getting to the finish line of a triathlon, marathon or long bike race is half mental. Having the will to get to the finish line takes incredible mental focus.

The preparation before the race is what allows you to keep pushing on, knowing that you have done what you need to do to prepare. When the surprises and challenges come along in a race, you find yourself better prepared to deal with them.

The Curveballs in Life

The purpose of a curveball is to surprise; to introduce something unexpected or something requiring a quick reaction or correction. Life is full of curveballs. How we deal with them defines us. Believe it or not preparation and planning ahead can help you deal with those unexpected curveballs in life.

Many people lost a lot of their retirement in one of the recent stock-market downturns, but not everyone did. Some people had some of their retirement in other vehicles, allowing them to weather the losses better. Others diversified streams of income to guard against one stream of income drying up. Also, people who prepare mentally for inevitable ups and downs in the stock market don't fall victim to it. Looking historically at stock market trends shows cyclical performance.

Speaking of the unexpected events and circumstances in our lives, perhaps it's not the curveball itself that surprises us, but the disappointment of falling short of our expectations. The curveball coming our way requires us to duck or dodge, altering our game plan, thus altering our expectations. We have to look at things differently, and sometimes the alternate path offered is a difficult one.

In my case, cancer and that surprise blockage that required two stents knocked me for a loop. Talk about curveballs! I thought of myself as invincible. I lived my life right. I did the right things from a health standpoint. Yet, I still had to deal with *two* curveballs.

Preparation includes setting goals. When you set small goals, you will achieve more. And the more positive experience in goals achievement we experience, the better the chances we'll have positive results in the future. Whatever goals you may set, know that you'll fail to achieve some, and that's okay. Failures, or the curveballs, are part of the process, and you should set aside your fear of them. Sometimes our goals don't lead to what we expected. Don't deprive yourself of a chance to take a loss. It's all part of the journey and we can learn from the tough situations in our lives.

Life is designed so that we look forward to the long-term and live short-term. We dream for the future and live in the present. You have the daily things you live for and do today with the hope for the retirement you always planned. The present can produce many difficult obstacles yet setting goals for the future provides long-term vision in our lives. We all need powerful, long-range goals to help us get past those short-term obstacles. Obstacles are just part of life. I love this quote by Karen Salmansohn, founder of NotSalmon.com. She is such a source of practical inspiration and strength.

"Give yourself time to heal from a challenge you've been dealt. Letting go of hurt doesn't happen overnight. It happens in slow, small forward (plus a few backwards at times). Be gentle and patient with yourself."

Reflective Questions

What area of your life have you ignored and not prepared for change? For example, what if you become ill or the status of your investments changes? What is your plan B?

How will being prepared help your peace of mind?

How will peace of mind impact the quality of your life?

Know Your Options

"Identify your problems, but give your power and energy to solutions."

– Tony Robbins

Looking back, I realized one small but huge difference between Bill and me regarding our outcomes with prostate cancer was early detection. My grandfather died of prostate cancer, so I have been extremely mindful and diligent about yearly PSA testing. Bill missed just one year of getting his PSA checked and it cost him his life.

Please note that I based this information on my personal research for my own treatment. You should not rely on it solely if you or a loved one faces prostate cancer. This is ONLY designed to help you ask the right questions.

The PSA test is controversial, as evidenced by the C grade recently assigned by the United States Preventive Services Task Force (USPSTF). The USPSTF, a national task force established in 1984, was created to make evidenced-based recommendations for clinical preventive services and health promotion, in order to aid primary care professionals, patients and families in deciding the appropriateness of a particular preventive service for an individual's needs. The Task Force assigns a letter grade of A, B, C, D or I to each recommendation based on the strength of the evidence and the advantages and disadvantages of the service under consideration.

In 2017, the USPSTF updated its recommendation on prostate cancer testing and upgraded its recommendation for the first time in 10 years to a C rating, meaning there's "at least a moderate certainty that the net benefit is small." The previous D rating labeled the PSA as doing "more harm than good," and strongly discouraged physicians from using the test for men at risk for the disease.

Jamie Bearse, CEO of ZERO - The End of Prostate Cancer said "While the improved recommendation is a step in the right direction, there is much work to do. We must undo a decade-long message that discouraged men from getting tested, and encourage men to talk to their doctor about their risks and the test. Unfortunately, the C rating is still insufficient and dangerous for high-risk men or men who – without testing – will develop aggressive or advanced disease."

The PSA test measures levels of protein released by the prostate, which may indicate the presence of cancer when elevated. But increased levels can also result from less serious medical conditions, like inflammation or infection, which is why many doctors are hesitant about the PSA test. Though not an absolute, it is a guide and benchmark, hence, the controversy.

Major evolution has occurred recently with prostate cancer screening, particularly with the use of Multiparametric (MP) MRI of the prostate to decide if there is a suspicion of prostate cancer (elevated PSA) needs a biopsy. The recent publications of a multi-site, multi-national PRECSION trial has further solidified the use of MRI as the best standard practice for a man with an elevated PSA. The increased specificity and locational information provided by MRI will mean that 30% of men with elevated PSAs can avoid a biopsy all together and those getting biopsies can get more accurate results The increased use of MRI and the use of adjunct PSA testing such as %free PSA, Prostate Health Index and the 4K Score blood tests (all more specific for prostate cancer than PSA) could help drive organization such as the USPSTF towards stronger advocacy for prostate cancer screening.

While working on figuring out how to fight cancer, I didn't just follow doctor's orders. Once I decided to fight the battle, I wanted to make sure I knew all my options and that I spent a significant amount of time exploring them. I believe an educated consumer is a smart consumer, especially when it comes to health care options. When life throws you a curveball, knowing your options is a first step to working through it.

Early Detection

As with any cancer, early detection is key and early detection tests for prostate cancer are:

☐ The PSA blood test or Prostate Specific Antigen (PSA) test: This test determines the level of PSA, a substance made by the prostate gland, in the blood. Levels of PSA can be higher in men with prostate cancer. Although PSA is mostly found in the semen, a small amount is also found in the blood. Most healthy men have levels under 4/ng/ml (nanograms per milliliter of blood. The chance of having prostate cancer goes up as the PSA level goes up. If your level falls between 4 and 10, your chance is over 33 percent. If above 10, your chance is over 50 percent. But some men with a PSA below 4 can also have prostate cancer. Also, age is a factor with the PSA.

Young men with a PSA in the 2.5ng/ml – 4ng/ml range should be alerted to the possibility of prostate cancer.

☐ Digital Rectal Exam (DRE): In this test, a physician inserts a finger into the rectum to feel the prostate for any irregular or firm areas that might be cancer. Though less effective than the PSA blood test in finding prostate cancer, it sometimes finds cancers in men with normal PSA levels. For this reason, it may be done as a part of prostate cancer screening.

☐ Multiparametric (MP) MRI: MPMRI is used when an elevated PSA or a positive DRE increases the suspicion for prostate cancer. The MRI is performed and it, and lesions within it are scored from 1 to 5. Men having scores of 1 and 2 can usually avoid biopsy while those with scores of 3-5 are usually biopsied using the MRI information fused to the ultrasound in real time to improve accuracy of sampling.

A caveat: No test is absolutely accurate!

As Craig Pynn said in his book, *Navigating the Realities of Prostate Cancer*[10], his cancer tricked his PSA mechanism,

---

[10] *Navigating the Realities of Prostate Cancer*, Craig Pynn

managing to remain undetected before it finally produced a visible symptom, blood in his urine. He felt no discomfort or pain. Craig was diagnosed with an aggressive tumor well on its way to being Stage 4 metastatic cancer had it not been caught in time, despite seven successive years of a 1.5 PSA.

With suspicion of cancer as a result of a PSA test, DRE or other factors, the doctor most likely will perform a biopsy. A biopsy is the only way to know for sure if cancer is present. During a biopsy, tissue from the prostate is removed and sent to the lab to see if it contains cancer cells.

Genomic testing is a type of specialized medical test done on cancerous tissue. These tests look at the makeup of the cancer and provide information about how the cancer may behave and the risk of spreading to other organs and parts of the body. The results can help with making a plan to manage prostate cancer. More than 50 percent of cases probably won't spread beyond the prostate.

Newly Diagnosed Prostate Cancer -- Questions for the Doctor

Here are the questions I asked my doctor and you should ask if you face a cancer diagnosis.

☐ What are my treatment options? Which do you recommend for me? Why?

☐ What are the expected benefits of each kind of treatment?

☐   What are the risks and possible side effects of each treatment? How can the side- effects be managed?

☐   What can I do to prepare for treatment?

☐   Will I need to be hospitalized? If so, for how long?

☐   What is the cost of treatment? Will my insurance cover it?

☐   How will treatment affect normal activities? Will it affect my sex life? Will I have urinary problems?

☐   Will I have bowel problems?

☐   Is a clinical trial an option?

With a prostate cancer diagnosis, you have many options. There is no one right answer.

Gleason Score and Staging

Once prostate cancer is confirmed, additional tests are done to learn the stage, and Gleason score, also known as the grade of the tumor. Grading using the Gleason score indicates how quickly the tumor will grow and spread. The grade describes the tumor based on how abnormal the cells look under the microscope:

☐ Gleason Grade Group 1 (Gleason 3+3= 6) - Tumor is well-differentiated, less aggressive and likely to grow more slowly

☐ Gleason Grade Group 2 and 3 (Gleason 3+4 and 4+3=)7 - Tumor is moderately differentiated, moderately aggressive, and likely to grow

☐ Gleason Grade Groups 4 and 5 (Gleason Sums of 8 or 9-10) - Tumor is poorly differentiated, highly aggressive and likely to grow fast and spread

If the biopsy indicates cancer, more tests can tell whether the cancer has spread and if so, how far, within the prostate and other parts of the body. This process called staging is very important because the treatment and outlook for recovery depend on the stage of the cancer. Below are the stages:

☐ Stage One - cancer is small and in the prostate only

☐ Stage Two - cancer is larger and may be in both lobes of the prostate

☐ Stage Three - cancer has spread beyond the prostate capsule into nearby structures such as the seminal vesicles

☐ Stage Four- cancer has spread to other organs such as the lymph nodes or the bone, also known as metastatic cancer

The best treatment for one man may not be the best for another. The right treatment depends on many factors, including:

☐ Age and life expectancy

☐ Gleason score of tumor

☐ Stage of prostate cancer

☐ Symptoms

☐ Any other serious health problems

☐ Personal feelings about the need to treat the cancer

☐ Personal feelings about the side effects common with each type of treatment

☐ The chance each type of treatment will cure the cancer or enhance the well being of the individual.

Here are some treatment options that I discovered.

Treatment - Early Stage Prostate Cancer

☐ Active Surveillance is the close monitoring of the status of the prostate cancer through regular office visits and repeat medical tests

☐ Surgery, known as a radical prostatectomy, is the removal of the entire prostate

☐ Radiation therapy destroys the cancer cells in the prostate while leaving the prostate in the body. It can be administered in two ways, externally and internally. External beam ration therapy is like an x-ray, but for a longer time. Each treatment lasts for a few minutes and is administered five times a week for approximately eight weeks. Internal radiation, called Brachytherapy, includes two types: permanent and temporary. Compared to external radiation, which requires five to eight weeks of daily treatments, convenience is a major advantage.

☐ Radiation brachytherapy. In Permanent (Low Dose Rate) Brachytherapy (LDR) a doctor or clinician implants radioactive (iodine-125 or palladium-103) seeds into the prostate gland using an ultrasound for guidance. A computer-generated treatment plan tailored for each patient determines the number of seeds and their placement.

Commonly, they place anywhere from 40 to 100 seeds and they remain in place permanently. After some months they become biologically inert (no longer useful). This technique allows for delivery of a high dose of radiation to the prostate with limited damage to surrounding tissues.

☐ Cryosurgery freezes the cells with cold metal probes. Cold gasses pass through the probes, which create ice balls that destroy the prostate gland.

☐ High Intensity focused ultrasound (HIFU) uses heat to kill prostate cancer cells. To administer, a doctor inserts an ultrasound probe into the rectum, then focuses beams of sound waves on cancerous portions of the gland. The heat technique is being used in several countries for treating localized prostate cancer.

Side Effects

☐ Incontinence - prostatectomy and radiation therapy can cause muscle damage that disrupts the way the bladder holds and discharges urine. Treatment depends on the severity of the condition.

☐ Erectile dysfunction

☐ Pain

☐ Depression

☐ Bowel injury

Treatment - Advanced Prostate Cancer

☐ **Hormone therapy**, also called androgen deprivation therapy

(ADT), lowers the testosterone level. Because prostate

cancer cells use testosterone as fuel, ADT starves the tumor cells.

Lowering androgen levels often makes the prostate cancer shrink or

grow more slowly. Hormone therapies do not kill prostate cancer,

but can provide relief from the symptoms and improve

the quality of life and extend survival. Hormone therapy can be

used at many points during the treatment, including with surgery

and radiation. Unfortunately, nearly all prostate cancers become

resistant to hormone therapy over time. Several types of hormone

therapy exist and they involve either surgery or the use of drugs to

lower the amount of testosterone or block the body's ability to use

androgen. One such treatment is with abiraterone; which blocks the

production of male hormones from the testis, adrenal glands and

prostate cancer cells itself. While this drug was traditionally added to men once their cancer progressed on hormonal therapy (became castrate resistant) new studies suggest that adding abiraterone early (in "dense" hormonal therapy) can prolong the survival of men with metastatic prostate cancer.

Side Effects

- Less sexual desire
- Erectile dysfunction
- Hot flashes
- Breast tenderness
- Bone thinning
- Anemia
- Decreased mental sharpness
- Loss of muscle mass
- Weight gain
- Fatigue
- Increased cholesterol
- Interference with diabetic meds for control of blood sugar

☐ **Immunotherapy** stimulates the immune system to kill cancer cells. For men with advanced disease, immunotherapy may be an option. For example, Provenge involves a treatment made by taking a man's blood cells and training them to destroy prostate cancer cells and then injecting them back into the man a few days later. Another type of immunotherapy is use of check point inhibitors like Pembrolizumab which can help take the "breaks" off the immune response and may have benefit in a select group of men with advanced prostate cancer (i.e. those who are found to have micro-satellite instability when genetics are assayed). Immunotherapy sometimes results in the immune system attacking healthy cells, which can cause side effects.

Side Effects

- Mouth sores
- Skin reactions.
- Flu-like symptoms
- High or low blood pressure
- Muscle aches
- Shortness of breath (trouble breathing)
- Swelling of legs (edema)
- Sinus congestion
- Headaches
- Weight gain from retaining fluid
- Diarrhea

- o Hormone changes
- o Cough

☐ **Chemotherapy** uses anti-cancer drugs (docetaxel) to kill cancer cells, usually administered intravenously. Like hormone therapy, chemo will not likely result in a cure. Though it fails to kill all the cancer cells, it may slow the cancer's growth and reduce the symptoms.

Side Effects

☐ Nausea

☐ Loss of appetite

☐ Hair loss

☐ Mouth sores

☐ Increased risk of infection (low white blood counts)

☐ Bleeding and bruising after minor injuries

☐ Tiredness (low red blood cell count)

☐ **Radiation for Bone Metastases** – If prostate cancer spreads to other parts of the body, it frequently spreads to the bone, which can cause pain, increased fractures and other problems. External radiation can be used to treat individual areas of the bone where the cancer has spread. Internal radiation, given as a shot, goes directly to the bone. It gives off strong energy to help kill off cancer cells, but damages healthy cells.

With a prostate cancer diagnosis you must consider many factors before choosing a course of action. These include age, overall health, goals for treatment and feelings about side effects. Some men can't imagine living with the side effects such as incontinence or impotence. Others are focused on getting rid of the cancer. If you are over 70 or have serious health problems, you might want to think of prostate cancer as a chronic disease because it will not lead to your death. Each man's case is unique and involves many factors. Any treatment will have side effects. Some may last for a few weeks or months, but others can be permanent.

Prostate cancer can come back many years after the initial treatment. This is called recurrence. Most doctors recommend PSA tests and digital rectal exams every 3-6 months for the first five years after treatment, and at least yearly after that.

What are Your Options?

You may have any number of problems in your life. Even if you don't have something as life-threatening as cancer, you could have financial, relationship or work issues you are dealing with.

Do you feel stranded, or like a victim with no place to turn? You are not a victim and you always have options. Let's say you are in a relationship with a really negative person to the point that it brings you down. How do you deal with it? Look at your options.

You have options from setting boundaries with the person when they start acting negative, to explaining how you feel when they act a certain way. Maybe you make it a point not to join in when they start criticizing people. You don't have to agree with or engage in anything they say. You have the choice to not contribute to the criticism. You could ask the person to refrain from their negative behavior. In some cases, physical distance from the person makes sense.

Maybe you work in a corporate job that keeps you stressed out much of the time. You may not be able to quit right away, but you can look at the other options you have. Even if you get laid off from a job, the result could push you to figure out huge life changes that make your life so much richer. You can always find more than one way to tackle an issue. Finding new ways to tackle a situation in your life can be concerning because you have to step out of your comfort zone into the unknown.

Knowing What You Want

When looking at treatment options know what you really want. When the doctor told me I had options for treatment that I should know about for dealing with cancer, I didn't want to hear them. I could not even consider the options. My brain had fogged over. I had not come to grips with the fact that I wanted to fight and live. Eventually, I knew that I needed and wanted to educate myself with the options. I knew I wanted the option that would have the least negative impact on my overall health. There is no one right answer when it comes to treating prostate cancer.

Maybe you work in a stressful situation because you want to provide for your family. That is an admirable motive, yet if you experience such stress that it impacts your health, or keeps you away from your family, maybe you need to consider other options.

Later in my technology career, I developed a passion for public safety and security. I wanted to make my community and the world a safer place by leveraging my background in technology. Knowing my options made a positive difference, for my employer, the world and me. I immersed myself in education through numerous citizen academies such as the FBI and Department of Public Safety, along with CERT (Citizens Emergency Response Team) and North Texas Crime Commission (ambassador).

Even with all that, I encountered bumps in my career path. The technology industry is fickle and ever changing, for both established companies and startups. I made mistakes by not knowing all my options. Eighty-five percent of all startups fail within the first five years. In some cases, I bought into the pitches about how great the startup and its services were, without conducting enough due diligence. I should have researched unique differentiators, sustainable advantage and what problem the company sought to solve. I should have made sure the company was not selling a solution looking for a problem or selling "smoke and mirrors." Also, I needed to figure out if the organization had the financial runway to succeed.

Knowing your options offers you choices. When I coached kids, I always wanted to teach them that making the right choices came from knowing all the options. The kids looked up to me as a role model and I strived to always set an example. I wanted to instill in them that no matter what challenge they faced or goal they wanted to achieve, to always look for the options.

There have been so many stories in the news of over-the-top parents and coaches related to youth sports teams, who wanted success so badly that they forgot about developing people into responsible human beings. I never wanted people to see me in that light. I always felt accountable for my actions and choices, and I wanted to teach kids to feel the same way.

To ensure my accountability to my own standards, I created *One Coach's Creed*, which can apply to life in general.

One Coach's Creed: Rules to Live By

I will never hesitate giving credit where credit is due. It's better to recognize a good performance than criticize a poor one.

I will look at each day as a new opportunity.

I will attack my daily work with boldness, enthusiasm and confidence, and I will persist until I achieve my goal.

If I fail, it is because I have chosen to fail.

By helping others to do their best and attain their goals, I help myself.

I recognize that each obstacle and defeat I must face and overcome sharpens my skill, strength, courage and understanding.

I will never forget how I got where I am today.

I consider sacrifice not as giving something up, but gaining something important toward the attainment of a personal goal.

I will live this day as if it is my last, not looking back to yesterday's mistakes or successes, and not worrying about what might come tomorrow.

I will not mix my personal problems with my work problems. I will work them out where they belong – at home and at work.

I will attempt to be honest and objective with myself and my players and try to give each individual the treatment he earns and deserves.

I believe that a man may make mistakes, but that he can't be considered a failure until he blames his mistakes on someone else.

By my actions and comments, I can influence my players and fellow workers, because one teaches by example.

I believe that winning and losing are in the guts and mind of a coach. Outwardly, he accepts success with equanimity, and defeat without criticism.

I will maintain a positive attitude. I will praise rather than put down, be hopeful rather than hopeless, be helpful instead of selfish, and be enthusiastic rather than complaining.

I will accept constructive guidance and suggestions when they are offered, and when I feel that I need help or support I will ask for it, not because I am weak or indecisive, but because I see a healthy dependence on others as a sign of strength and independence.

Whatever you do in life, you always have options and choices. The more you take responsibility for knowing your options and making the right choices, the richer your life. None of us are victims unless we choose to be. That does not mean that bad things that are out of our control will not happen. A drunk driver might smash into your car. If you survive, you have the choice of how to live the rest of your life. I found a great story about this in Hal Elrod's book *The Miracle Morning*. He tells a great story of his life and choosing to live and survive in the face of trauma.

What options do you have for your life and major decisions? You always have various ways to deal with anything in your life. Always look at your options for dealing with any situation. You will be amazed at how it empowers you. Live your best life now! Be an IRONMAN of life!

Reflective Questions

What do you face in your life, where you need to explore options?

What shifts in your attitude do you need to make to explore the options?

Live Beyond Yourself

"I profoundly feel that the art of living is the art of giving. You're fulfilled in the moment of giving, of doing something beyond yourself."

— Laurance Rockefeller, Businessman

As I have mentioned, to become an IRONMAN, you must be somewhat self-absorbed and self-centered. Training requires great time-management skills. The typical personality of an IRONMAN is driven and goal-oriented in all aspects of life. Those who struggle with that balance can't seem to balance all aspects of their life.

To quote four-time IRONMAN Champion Chrissie Wellington, inducted into the IRONMAN Hall of Fame in the Fall of 2017, "We talk about 'I' in this sport, but it's really about 'WE'. We do a selfish sport; sometimes we need to do something selfless."

For me, self-less meant racing for a bigger cause. As Chrissie said, and as I've mentioned before, training and competing in IRONMAN races is a lifestyle. For many years others around me had to adjust their lives and support me in that. After surviving cancer and racing for a cause, to inspire others, my focus and motivation changed.

The imbalance reminds me of a child striving to become a world-class athlete. They miss out on so many life and childhood experiences. With an adult training for an IRONMAN, the negative ramifications and impact on those around the athlete can prove enormous. In a sense, family and friends must commit to the sport as much as the athlete.

Initially, when I registered for IRONMAN, Lake Placid, 2016 I had a two-fold motivation. First, I wanted to set a crazy goal to strive for, to get beyond my cancer and recovery. The second was to honor the memory of my friend Bill Rollings.

At that point, I still had not shared my plight with anyone outside my immediate circle. I kept my suffering inside. When I decided to "come out of the closet" with my battle in March 2016, suddenly it mushroomed into something much bigger than me. I wanted to compete for more than Tom's self-satisfaction. I wanted to race for a cause and cancer patients everywhere around the world. I had never been in a situation where so many people followed me. I had become a beacon of hope and inspiration for cancer patients around the world. The hope and inspiration even extended to others with life challenges other than cancer.

On the day of my surgery, my surgeon gave me a cool looking wristband. It said ZERO End Prostate Cancer. I only saw it as a neat slogan, nothing more. But, I've never taken it off. I see it as a constant reminder of what I have survived. I drew strength from it while training and racing. It is a tangible reminder of my journey and mission to help others.

In early 2016 I googled ZERO and learned what it stood for. Their mission and vision immediately resonated with me.

Mission

"ZERO — The End of Prostate Cancer is the leading national nonprofit with the mission to end prostate cancer. ZERO advances research, improves the lives of men and families, and inspires action."

Vision

"Imagine a future with zero prostate cancer deaths and an end to pain and suffering. Our vision is Generation ZERO – the first generation of men free from prostate cancer . . ."

This is now my vehicle for making a difference. After more due diligence, I joined the ZERO Endurance Team. The team's slogan is "Add meaning to your miles." That ignited a passion in me that still burns intensely to this day. I want to put an end to the suffering caused by prostate cancer.

My mission is to get the world one step closer to Generation ZERO – the first generation of men free from prostate cancer. Donations to ZERO fund research, patient financial assistance, early detection, and educational programs. One of the reasons I've so passionately embraced this philanthropic effort is that over 90 cents of every donated dollar goes to program expenses. That is an amazing financial metric!

Here is more information about ZERO, from their website at zerocancer.org.

"Most people don't know that a watershed moment for prostate cancer was inspired by breast cancer. In 1996, several groups of concerned patients, physicians, and advocates came together to create the National Prostate Cancer Coalition. Modeled after the National Breast Cancer Coalition, this new organization was formed to stand up for men and their families impacted by prostate cancer and become a political force for a cure.

The first challenge was to create public awareness and a collective voice for the prostate cancer movement. We brought the face of prostate cancer to Congress with testimony from survivors and those who lost loved ones to the disease, spearheading the Department of Defense's Prostate Cancer Research Program. We championed strategic alliances with national and local organizations and politicians to protect critical government funds for prostate cancer research. We pioneered free mobile prostate cancer screening across the nation through our Drive Against Prostate Cancer program, testing more than 130,000 at risk men and alerting them to potentially life-saving information.

As the prostate cancer landscape has evolved, so have we. Today, we are the destination for taking action to end prostate cancer and making prostate cancer research a national priority. With a new name, ZERO – The End of Prostate Cancer, we are still on the front lines in Washington, DC and grassroots communities to provide much needed programs that positively impact the lives of both men at risk and men suffering from this disease. We're providing men and families with educational resources and funding promising research for improved early detection options. Our mantra to support, educate, and activate is mobilizing a like-minded, passionate, and multigenerational army of advocates across the country to end prostate cancer.

Whether you are a 40-year-old father of three young children in the prime of your life or a 65-year-old excited to enjoy your retirement and spend time with your grandchildren, the face of prostate cancer can look very different. What unites us all is our steadfast commitment to eliminate the pain and suffering and create Generation ZERO – the first generation of men free from prostate cancer."[11]

Surviving the Physical Struggle

Getting to the start line at Lake Placid in 2016 was in my reality the finish line, a celebration of life. That race at Lake Placid was the hardest physical challenge of my life, even more challenging than the Mountain Man Winter Triathlon ("Winter Ironman"). The three disciplines, in order, were cross-country skiing, snowshoe running and speed skating.

Let me give some context to the difficulty of the Mountain Man. I found the course description most intimidating. "It is one of the most brutal tests of winter mountaineering the human body is capable of performing in one day with elevation changes of over 14,000. Contestants should be prepared to spend the entire race in the unpredictable weather patterns that the winter mountain climate has to offer."

In addition, I had never cross-country skied or worn snowshoes. So, I improvised. To learn how to cross country ski, I spent hours on a NordicTrack machine. Subsequently, Nordic Track became my sponsor. I utilized muscle-specific training for snowshoe running, by running in a shallow pool and working out on a Stairmaster with 30 pounds strapped to my body. Fortunately, I knew how to skate. In subsequent years, I utilized speed skating

---

[11] ZEROcancer.org

coach Rob Blair (His sister Bonnie is a five-time Olympic gold medalist, the most decorated woman in Winter Olympic history and "Sports Illustrated" Sportswoman of the Year).

With Rob's coaching and converting from hockey to speed skates, I improved to 7th overall in the speed skating leg. This helped me to a Top 25 finish in my 6th and final year of competing in the Mountain Man. Not bad for someone previously told that "no way a flatlander from south of the Mason-Dixon line could even finish." I found The Mountain Man was quite a challenge, but it paled to racing an IRONMAN only 14 months after prostate cancer surgery.

Even though I struggled mightily at Lake Placid, finishing 22 minutes before the midnight cutoff, and wondering if I could even compete at Kona eleven weeks later, something kept driving me forward. Racing for a cause for the benefit of others got me over that finish line. And as you can imagine, the race at Lake Placid had a very different meaning for me.

During those downs at Lake Placid, I thought about how lucky I felt to compete. The blue ZERO wristband that my surgeon gave me after the operation has served as a constant reminder of who I'm racing for and my mission to make a difference. That wristband helped me power through at Lake Placid. I had a lot of self-induced pressure at Lake Placid. In the past, if I quit a race (DNF), nobody would have really cared. Now I had people who supported me in my fund-raising efforts of over $32,000 for ZERO. They were watching.

A sign that I saw along the IRONMAN Coeur d'Alene course in 2007 always stuck with me: "Pain is temporary. Quitting is forever." This quote resonates with me more than ever now. I have a purpose bigger than myself.

On top of racing for a cause, Lake Placid has a very special place in my heart, part of the reason I selected it for my long-term goal in beating cancer. Lake Placid hosted the 1980 Olympics' drama of "The Miracle on Ice," the USA hockey team's upset of Russia. *Sports Illustrated* labeled it the number one sport's moment of the 20th century.

The finish line of IRONMAN sits on the Olympic Oval, across from the "Miracle" Arena. A great hockey fan since my childhood, finishing there, was certainly one of the most significant moments of my life. Herb Brooks, legendary coach of that miracle hockey team told his players just before the start of the game, "You were born to be a player. You were meant to be here. This moment is yours." Goose bumps. Beat the Russians!

The Final IRONMAN

An amazing thing happened when I participated in my last IRONMAN. I raced Kona 2.5 hours faster than Lake Placid. Lauren almost missed me getting to the finish line, because of how much my time improved. How special to have her at the finish line cheering me on. The significance of the moment was huge. We had fought the cancer battle together. Her encouragement, like a beacon of light and strength, helped lead me through the ordeal.

Serving a Higher Cause

Since that Kona race in 2016, I have continued in my contribution to fighting prostate cancer, and it has taken me to a different level of life. It's a great feeling to give back to help others who face what I faced.

ZERO Cancer Summit

In 2017 and 2018, I attended the ZERO Cancer Summit on Capitol Hill, as a scholarship recipient and advocate. We met with members of Congress and the Senate. One of the outcomes was a historic victory for prostate cancer research. The Department of Defense (DOD)'s Prostate Cancer Research Program (PCRP) received its first increase of $10 Million in funding in over a decade and is now funded at $100 Million.

I never expected the therapeutic benefit of the Summit. For the first time, I met and heard from other prostate cancer survivors. They shared their emotions and their stories. Amazingly, the Summit made a difference in the fight against prostate cancer, and it helped me so much, emotionally. I learned a very valuable lesson.

You cannot experience cancer in isolation because the feeling of aloneness can swiftly overtake you.

Congressionally Directed Medical Research Programs (CDMRP)

In the fall of 2017, ZERO nominated me to participate as a Consumer Reviewer Panelist for the DOD's CDMRP. As a Consumer Reviewer I participated as a full voting member, (along with prominent scientists) at meetings to help determine the allocation of the $90 Million appropriated by Congress for Fiscal Year 2017 for the Prostate Cancer Research Program (PCRP). CDMRP asks Consumer Reviewers to represent the collective view of patients by preparing comments on the impact of the research on issues such as diagnosis, treatment, and quality of life. Since 1996 Consumer advocates and scientists have worked together in this unique partnership to evaluate the scientific merit of research applications.

Colonel Wanda L. Salzer, M.D., Director of the CDMRP said, "The Consumer Reviewers on each panel are instrumental in helping the scientists understand the patient's perspective and provide valuable insight into the potential impact of the proposed project. They bring with them a sense of urgency and remind us all, of the human element involved in medical research."

Scientists applying propose to conduct innovative research focused on the elimination of death from prostate cancer and enhancing the well being of men experiencing the impact of prostate cancer. The PCRP fills important gaps not addressed by other funding agencies by supporting groundbreaking, high-risk, high-gain research while encouraging out-of-the-box thinking.

To date, $1.53 billion has been granted for prostate cancer via the CDMRP. I felt so honored to be a Consumer Reviewer. I am humbled and excited to know that I have served to make an impact in the battle against cancer, and/or enhanced the well being of men experiencing the disease.

A hallmark of the CDMRP review process program is the Moment of Silence (MOS) to mark the beginning of the meeting plenary. The MOS is a three-minute speech that sets the tone for the entire program. The MOS reminded all the participants (200+ scientists) of our purpose. Another honor came my way when officials asked me to deliver the MOS. Despite being outside my comfort zone (again), it was totally worth it to stand up and speak for the sake of others.

Baylor, Scott & White Medical Center

I currently volunteer at the Baylor, Scott & White Cancer Health & Wellness Center in Plano, Texas. I lead exercise classes for people recovering from cancer. Physical fitness supports total health, both physical and mental. With the program, we encourage patients to be active as they recover. I also advocate for cancer patients who come through the center. Dealing with cancer is an emotional roller coaster. People who have not walked through it, don't always understand. Sometimes health care providers seem calloused to the challenges someone faces. As an example, the doctor who performed my surgery struck me as very cold. To him, I was just a number. It would have been nice to feel like he understood my fear and uncertainty.

According to the American Cancer Society the lifetime risk of developing cancer is 1 in 2 for men and 1 in 3 for women. The Center caters to cancer survivors. When is someone a "cancer survivor?"

The Center's philosophy is: "Survivor from the time of diagnosis, through treatment, and beyond." The Center is a home for cancer survivors and families. In addition to the gym, the Center includes a resource center and educational rooms. Programs include exercise, education, art, therapy and healthy cooking demonstrations.

I also supported the ZERO 5K Run/Walk Series, which helps bring awareness to ZERO and its mission. The ZERO Prostate Cancer Run/Walk series is the premier program of ZERO with 40 events across the country. Advocates come together for a Run/Walk, to raise funds and share hope to declare one number: ZERO. Participants make a real difference in the lives of men and families fighting prostate cancer, for example, funding research for a test to distinguish aggressive from slow-growing disease, to providing educational and support resources to at-risk men in the community. Participants drive ZERO's mission to end prostate cancer and have a direct impact in their local communities. In 2017, the ZERO 5K Run/Walk raised $3.5 million and hosted 20,000 participants.

As Lauren said, "If I can save one life while I still have mine, this journey will have purpose."

I find my volunteer work at the Cancer Health & Wellness Center so gratifying. When the people I work with hear my story, they realize that they too can hope. Some of the people I work with may not beat cancer, but amazingly, each time I do this volunteer work, people light up when they see me, because I offer them hope. I am so humbled by the fact that my experience brings hope to others. The tough battle I fought will make a difference in the world for others.

As fellow CDMRP reviewer Tony Minter said, "I aspire to inspire before I expire."

How Does Living Beyond Yourself Impact You?

How can you live a life of significance beyond yourself? I hope that my story will inspire you to look beyond yourself, to see how your life can have a positive impact on others. Recent history offers us a number of people to inspire us, who lived for purposes beyond themselves to make a great impact on the planet. Nelson

Mandela, Martin Luther King, and St. Theresa of Calcutta (Mother Teresa) come to mind. I'm sure you can think of many others.

What keeps people healthy and happy into their 80s or 90s? They live for a bigger purpose. They have a vision and mission for their existence.

I feel fortunate to have a mission to help others; to help them through the battles I survived and the emotional ups and downs of my journey. It's the IRONMAN race of life!

It's Not about the Tattoo

I never liked tattoos, but then again, I never thought I would have cancer. Two days after returning from the World Championships in Hawaii in 2016, I got "inked" with a big and bold M-dot on my calf. After getting comfortable with one tattoo, I decided to get another with another brand that fires my passion, ZERO – The End of Prostate Cancer.

According to the *Wall Street Journal*, the M-dot, or IRONMAN logo, is the second most popular brand tattooed on bodies, right after the Harley-Davidson. The common denominator for these two very different brands is passion.

Why did I get the tattoos? To advertise my passion for IRONMAN and ZERO and my mission to help wipe out prostate cancer. They are great conversation starters. Though I have completed eleven IRONMANs, facing death in the face was the most unnerving situation I have ever faced. My life mantra is embodied in the very definition of IRONMAN found on their website.

Anything is Possible

"IRONMAN is a statement of excellence, passion and commitment. It is a test of physical toughness and mental strength. IRONMAN is about persevering, enduring and being a part of something larger than ourselves. It shows the heights that can be achieved when we push beyond our boundaries and go the distance."[12]

It really isn't about the tattoos, but they are strong symbols that represent all I am. I got "inked" to always remember what I have survived, even though I will never forget. I am so proud to wear both brands. They are my identity, and a representation of my mission in life.

I sincerely hope that my story has given you the inspiration to fight any challenge you have and look beyond yourself and your circumstances. The unexpected and challenges in life's journey make you stronger and often prepare you to carry out your mission in life.

---

[12] IRONMAN Website: http://www.ironman.com/#ixzz56kkc5lpF

Reflective Questions

How can you live beyond yourself?

What gift, talent or ability can you use to encourage and support others?

How will significance in terms of contribution to human kind impact your quality of life?

What's Next?

I raced my last IRONMAN at the 2016 World Championship at Kona Hawaii. What a race to be your last! The euphoria of crossing the finish line was quickly replaced by "what's next?" I had a bit of an emotional letdown, because I had no future goal. I had invested so much time in training and forgoing other activities, but now what? After previous races, I looked for the next challenge.

The reason I competed in the World Championship at Kona in 2016 was very personal but it also gave me the platform to share my message. I continue to leverage this experience to bring higher awareness to the prevalence and risk of having prostate cancer. I've made it my life's mission to share my story about the disease and stress the importance of screening and early detection for any cancer. I want to eliminate this disease, and help improve the quality of life of those who currently live with prostate cancer.

2018 American Cancer Society Facts and Figures Implications for Prostate Cancer

It is widely reported that cancer mortality rates have dropped; down nearly two percent since 2015. On the surface, it's a good step toward minimizing the pain and suffering endured by many families, but one important detail that the media and medical advisors have glossed over is that prostate cancer deaths will jump 10 percent in 2018, the largest jump in prostate cancer deaths in a decade, according to the American Cancer Society[13].

The numbers speak for themselves

Fact	2017	2018
Estimated new cases	161,360	164,690
Estimated deaths	26,730	29,430
A new diagnosis every . . .	3.3 minutes	3.2 minutes
A man will die every . . .	20 minutes	18 minutes

---

[13] AmericanCancerSociety.org

What's Next?

How You Can Help

All the net proceeds from this book will go to prostate cancer research and education. In addition, I would appreciate your support by making a tax-deductible contribution to ZERO; www.zerocancer.org/tomhulsey. ZERO The End of Prostate Cancer is a 501c3 charity recognized with four stars by Charity Navigator, and a Better Business Bureau member.

Reflective Questions

What's next for you? Do you need to look forward and beyond yourself?

How will taking the next steps in your life make it richer?

What will you do today to contribute to a cause beyond yourself?

The Winning Attitude that Saved My Life

What's Next?

Made in the USA
Columbia, SC
30 November 2018